Health Services Research:
Avoiding common pitfalls

610.72

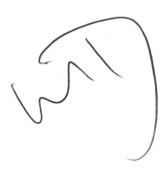

Other titles in the *Hospital Medicine* monograph series:

Vignettes for the MRCOG, volume 1 edited by Roy G Farquarson
Vignettes for the MRCOG, volume 2 edited by Roy G Farquarson
Vignettes for the MRCOG, volume 3 edited by Roy G Farquarson
Clinical Governance: One year on edited by Alastair P Scotland

Health Services Research:
Avoiding common pitfalls
Hospital Medicine monograph

edited by
Huw T.O. Davies

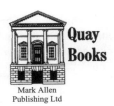

Quay
Books

Mark Allen
Publishing Ltd

300·72
DOV

Quay Books Division, Mark Allen Publishing Ltd
Jesses Farm, Snow Hill, Dinton, Wiltshire, SP3 5HN

British Library Cataloguing-in-Publication Data
A catalogue record is available for this book

© Mark Allen Publishing Ltd 2001
ISBN 1 85642 195 3

TC00462

Printed in the UK by Bath Press, Bath

Contents

List of contributors

Iain K Crombie, James Mackenzie Professor of Epidemiology and Public Health, University of Dundee

Huw TO Davies, Professor of Health Care Policy and Management, University of St Andrews

Julian PL Davis, Research Fellow, University of Dundee

Aileen R Neilson, Senior Scientist in Health Economics, Health Econ AG, Switzerland

Alison E Powell, Researcher in Health Care Management, University of St Andrews

Manouche Tavakoli, Lecturer in Applied Economics, University of St Andrews

Richard Thomson, Professor of Epidemiology and Public Health, University of Newcastle

Fiona LR Williams, Senior Lecturer in Epidemiology and Environmental Health, University of Dundee

Foreword

Huw Davies

For many health care professionals, busy working lives leave little time for an active involvement with research projects. Yet all health care professionals are enjoined to engage with the research evidence pertinent to their service areas. It is to assist such an engagement that this book has been addressed.

Health care, like many other public services (Davies, Nutley *et al*, 2000), has spent the last few decades embracing the 'evidence-based' paradigm. This natural science-led perspective is not the only way in which health care can be studied (Pope and Mays, 1995; Alderson, 1998), but nonetheless this predominantly positivistic approach — based on measurement and the search for generalisable 'laws' — has dominated the mainstream literature.

Health services research is the broad church that seeks to provide an empirical basis for health care delivery. It has many definitions (see *Box p. xii* for a few examples, and Crombie and Davies, 1996 for a fuller discussion) but, in essence, it explores the interface where people (as patients, as clients, as carers) meet services (usually delivered by health care professionals). The past few decades have seen a phenomenal growth in the availability of empirical work that explores this interface, asking such questions as:

- what are patients like?
- how are they diagnosed?
- what happens to them over time?
- how do they engage with health services?
- how should they be managed within the system?

As more and more research has become available, and as accounts have emerged about the gaps between that evidence and regular practice (Antman, Lau *et al*, 1992; Lau, Antman *et al*, 1992; Ketley and Woods, 1993), health care professionals are enjoined to integrate up-to-date findings in their work. This imperative to 'consult the evidence' has embraced not just doctors, but also nurses and the many professions allied to medicine. Beyond this, policy makers, health care planners, managers and patient advocates all frequently cast (at least some of) their activities within an evidence-based framework. Research has moved from being an arcane activity of the few, to a part of the day-to-day rhetoric of the many (even politicians are tempted to embrace its charms).

At the same time awareness has grown that not all research — even that published in the best of journals — is necessarily particularly informative (Fowkes *et al*, 1991; Thomas *et al*, 1998). Carrying out high quality research that provides accurate and trustworthy findings is no mean feat. Indeed, much published research is small scale, inconclusive, or even deeply flawed; the findings may mislead as well as enlighten. Yet how are health care professionals and other interested parties to separate substantive work from that which, while perhaps interesting, offers poor empirical justification for its conclusions? New skills of critical engagement and research interpretation are needed.

Critical appraisal is the interrogation of research to enable a clearer appreciation of the evidence it may have to offer. It is, in essence, a dialogue conducted between the appraiser and the appraised. At its simplest this involves asking questions about how the research was designed, implemented, analysed and interpreted. These questions can begin at the broadest of levels, for example:

- what was the basic research design, and was it suitable?
- were control groups included, and should they have been?
- was the study big enough?

Other questions may be highly technical and detailed:

- were the assumptions underlying the statistical testing violated?
- does the Cronbach's Alpha indicate sufficient internal consistency?

These interrogation skills, which this book addresses, are not currently widespread in health care. One of the advantages of approaching appraisal in a multi-level and structured way is that anyone can learn a few basic questions that can lay bare study flaws and open the way to more realistic evaluation.

There is no shortage of texts that seek to teach research methods for those who wish to develop research studies (see, for example, Hulley and Cummings, 1988; Polgar and Thomas, 1991; Sackett, Haynes *et al*, 1991; Lowe, 1993; Crombie and Davies, 1996;

Bowling, 1997). This book takes a rather different tack: it aims to provide the uninitiated with an easy route to developing the knowledge, skills and confidence to try critical appraisal for themselves. This ground is not untravelled, and many other helpful texts cover similar themes with varying emphases (Crombie, 1996; Greenhalgh, 1997; Sackett, Richardson *et al*, 1997; Greenhalgh and Donald, 2000). This entry-level text should be seen as complementary to the many other (text and web-based) resources in this area, and pointers to other sources are always given within each chapter.

This book takes the view that while knowing how to carry out research is valuable, for many busy professionals a more realistic expectation is that they should be able to read, understand and critique published research. The text, which gathers together a series of articles that appeared in *Hospital Medicine* in 1998–2001, provides guidance to a wide array of the most widely used research methods. Underlying each chapter is the view that many of the pitfalls that trap unwary researchers make it through to print and are commonly encountered in the published literature. Each piece focuses on explaining these flaws and providing simple ways to ease their identification. While the chapters are presented in an (arguably) logical sequence, each is in fact self-standing and they can be consulted in any order. Cross-referencing between chapters and to the best of an extensive literature provides ready routes to further information. Key points summarise each chapter; the virtues of brevity and simplicity are guiding principles.

The material presented is in two sections. In *Section I* some of the basic building blocks of research are introduced. Issues that arise in measurement, sampling and chance variability are all elaborated, as they arise whatever the basic research designs employed. Some of the interpretation difficulties are discussed, for example, separating association from causation, or interpreting reported costs and benefits. These again have widespread significance. In *Section II*, issues in research design are tackled separately for most of the main research methods. Surveys, trials, cohorts and case-control studies are all described and assessed for the common ways that they may be ill-designed. Finally, broader issues are addressed, such as those involved in systematic reviews, decision-analytic studies or even clinical audit.

An old adage (provenance unknown to this author) holds that, 'it ain't so much that I don't know, but that I know so much that ain't so'. Armed with the questions elaborated in this text, it is the hope that readers of the research literature will be better inoculated against the acquisition of such unsubstantiated or erroneous knowledge.

Box: Health services research

Broadly defined

❖ All strategic and applied research concerned with the health needs of the community as a whole, including the provision of services to meet those needs (House of Lords Select Committee on Science and Technology, 1988).

More specifically

❖ Research relating to the effectiveness of clinical practice, the dispersal and use of existing knowledge, and the contribution of medical interventions to the health status of individuals and populations (Drummond, Crump *et al*, 1992).

❖ The identification and quantification of health care needs, and the quantitative study of the provision and use of health services to meet them (The Wellcome Trust, 1993).

❖ The evaluation of the adequacy, effectiveness, and efficiency of medical care, including assessments of the need for medical care and of professional and public attitudes (Fowkes, Garraway *et al*, 1991).

References

Alderson P (1998) Theories in health care and research: The importance of theories in health care. *Br Med J* **317**: 1007–10

Antman EM, Lau JB, Kupelnick B, Chalmers TC (1992) A comparison of results of meta-analyses of randomized control trials and recommendations of clinical experts. *J Am Med Assoc* **268**: 240–8

Bowling A (1997) *Research Methods in Health: investigating health and health services.* Open University Press, Buckingham

Crombie IK (1996) *The Pocket Guide to Critical Appraisal.* BMJ Publishing, London

Crombie IK, Davies HTO (1996) *Research in Health Care: design, conduct and interpretation of health services research.* John Wiley & Sons, Chichester

Davies HTO, Nutley SM, Smith PC, eds (2000) *What works? Evidence-based policy and practice in public services.* The Policy Press, Bristol

Drummond MF, Crump BJ, Little VA (1992) Funding research and development in the NHS. *Lancet* **339**: 230–1

Fowkes FGR, GarrawayWM, Sheehy CK(1991) The quality of health services research in medical practice in the United Kingdom. *J Epidemiol Community Health* **45**: 102–6

Greenhalgh T (1997) *How to Read a Paper: the basics of evidence-based medicine.* BMJ Publishing Group, London

Greenhalgh T, Donald A (2000) *Evidence-based Health Care Workbook.* BMJ Publishing, London

House of Lords Select Committee on Science and Technology (1988) *Priorities in Medical Research. Volume I — Report.* HMSO, London

Hulley SB, Cummings SR, eds (1988) *Designing Clinical Research.* Williams & Wilkins, Baltimore

Ketley D, Woods KL (1993) Impact of clinical trials on clinical practice: example of thrombolysis for acute myocardial infarction. *Lancet* **342**: 891–4

Lau J, Antman EM, Jimenez-Silva J, Kupelnick B, Mosteller F, Chalmers TC (1992) Cumulative meta-analysis of therapeutic trials for myocardial infarction. *New Engl J Med* **327**: 248–54

Lowe D (1993) *Planning for Medical Research: A practical guide to research methods.* Astraglobe Limited, Middlesbrough

Polgar S, Thomas SA (1991) *Introduction to Research in the Health Sciences.* Churchill Livingstone, Edinburgh

Pope C, Mays N (1995) Qualitative Research: Reaching the parts other methods cannot reach: an introduction to qualitative methods in health and health services research. *Br Med J* **311**: 42–45

Sackett DL, Haynes RB, Guyatt GH, Tugwell P (1991) *Clinical Epidemiology: A Basic Science for Clinical Medicine.* Little, Brown and Company, Boston, Massachusetts

Sackett DL, Richardson WS, Rosenberg W, Haynes RB (1997) *Evidence-based Medicine: how to practice and teach EBM.* Churchill Livingstone, London

The Wellcome Trust (1993) *Health Services Research, Other grants for support of research in health services research and clinical epidemiology.* The Wellcome Trust, London

Thomas T, Fahey T, Somerset M (1998) The content and methodology of research papers published in three United Kingdom primary care journals. *Br J Gen Pract* **48**: 1229–32

Introducing critical appraisal

Huw Davies

All health care professionals are being encouraged to use research evidence more in developing their clinical practice. To do this they need to inculcate the skills of 'critical appraisal'. Such skills involve assessing the appropriateness of research designs for answering clinical questions, critiquing the quality of the data gathered in individual studies, and assessing the implications of research findings.

All health care professionals are enjoined to engage with research evidence in delivering their services. Health care managers need to be able to understand the implications of research for service re-configuration and development. Indeed, as health services research has burgeoned over the past decade, many more health care professionals are becoming actively involved in research projects large and small. While not everybody within health care needs to be a researcher, the great majority need to be able to read and understand research, and apply the findings in practice.

Critical appraisal is a structured way of reading research reports, which lays bare their key features. As these are scrutinised, the reader can ask whether the basic design is appropriate to the issues in hand, how well the study was carried out, and what are the implications of the findings. The critical appraisal approach involves asking a series of questions as a means of interrogating written research reports. These questions structure our thinking and greatly speed the task of reading and assimilating published research.

Beginning with a question

Research aimed at clinical practice can fall into a number of distinct categories. First, research studies may help to elucidate the causes or risk factors for disease. Second, research may describe the natural history of disease, allowing some estimates of likely prognosis if the condition is untreated. Third, research may help to appraise the usefulness of some kind of test for a disease. And finally, research may help inform on the likely benefits of interventions. The crucial point is that different research designs are differently able to provide reliable guidance in each of these areas. Thus the first key question to ask is what do I want to know and what research design is best able to provide this information?

The right design

Different research designs address different clinical questions. Exploring disease aetiology is done using either cohort studies or case-control studies depending on whether the disease of interest is common with early onset or rare with a long lag between exposure to pathogen and onset of disease. Although cross-sectional surveys are sometimes used to explore associations with disease they are a weak and inadequate design for this purpose.

In describing prognosis, cohort studies provide the best basis for estimating the likelihood of specific outcomes, with qualitative studies providing richer descriptions of these outcomes and their meaning to patients (see *Chapter 16*). Simple surveys of sufferers are again inadequate for understanding natural history as we have no way of knowing who has been omitted from the sample (deaths for example, or those who have recovered).

It is in appraising diagnostic or screening tests that cross-sectional studies may be helpful — so long as there is a 'gold standard' against which the new test is compared (in blinded fashion) and a full spectrum of individuals are included. Such studies cannot address the issue of whether or not better diagnostic information will improve health outcomes. For this, longitudinal studies are required.

Assessing the impact of interventions on health outcomes is the area where most methodological development has been seen. To answer questions of whether specific treatments or whole programmes of care are better than the alternatives requires very careful attention to design. Although cohort and case-control studies have been used to suggest therapeutic benefit, without doubt the most appropriate designs are large, well-conducted randomised control trials with other safeguards against bias such as blinding. Better still are systematic reviews with meta-analysis of several randomised control trials. Before-and-after studies, or uncontrolled designs, may suggest fruitful areas for more rigorous study but do not of themselves usually provide definitive guidance.

The design done right

All research designs are prone to bias during their design, implementation, analysis or interpretation. Observational studies (such as surveys, cohort studies or case-control designs) are particularly susceptible to confounding (*Chapter 7*), but have other potential pitfalls as well which are explored in subsequent chapters (*Chapters 10–13*). For example, in assessing prognosis, a crucial consideration is that any cohort study has gathered an inception cohort and has achieved full follow-up.

Controlled trials have evolved in sophistication over the past 50 years in an attempt to eliminate bias. Blinding (single, double or even triple), intention-to-treat analyses, and careful assessment of balance at baseline are all now key features of rigorous studies (*Chapters 5 and 14*). Systematic reviews have also now developed their own tradition of rigour and have taken over from the traditional narrative review (*Chapter 15*). Assessing the implications of chance remains essential for all of these research designs (Brennan and Croft, 1994; and *Chapter 6*).

For each of the major research designs there is now a wealth of literature which develops step-by-step guides or checklists for the appraisal of published research. To go with these checklists, several useful texts also provide considerable exploration of the key ideas underlying critical appraisal and evidence-based practice (Crombie, 1996; Greenhalgh, 1997; Sackett *et al*, 1997). Further guidance can be found in the Users' Guides developed by the Evidence-Based Medicine Working Group (EBMWG) led by Gordon Guyatt; formerly published in *JAMA* these are now available on the Internet (www.cche.net).

Assessing local relevance

Once any given study has been assessed as offering trustworthy evidence (ie. good **internal** validity), we turn to the question of whether the evidence will generalise to other settings or indeed particularise to our own setting (ie. the question of **external** validity).

Such questions are less one of checklists and more those of judgements. Four key considerations arise. First, how similar are the patients in the study to patients seen elsewhere and locally? Second, are the interventions described readily replicable in other settings? Third, are the outcomes described the key outcomes of local interest? And finally, are there features of the setting where the research was carried out which suggest that the findings would not transfer well to other areas?

It is clear that none of the four questions above have simple answers. Yet consideration of each provides some structure around which to investigate the question of transferability of research findings from one setting to another.

Assessing the implications

It can be difficult at times to assess the importance of new research findings for clinical practice. Again, some simple questions can help clarify. For diagnostic tests, the key question is: will the findings from the test provide sufficient information to inform a treatment strategy? For studies of prognosis, we are concerned about how patients feel about the range of possible outcomes and their attendant likelihood; and for studies of therapies the key issue is whether the potential benefits outweigh the possible harm. Information from several research studies may need to be combined with the individual patient's own preferences to develop a clinical management strategy.

Thus evidence on its own is incomplete. It needs to be particularised to individual patients. This process draws upon the collective experience and wisdom of clinicians known as 'clinical expertise'. It is this integration of best evidence with patient preferences facilitated by clinical expertise which is the hallmark of evidence-based practice. This integration cannot readily be reduced to a series of checklists: it draws on professional tacit knowledge accumulated through experience.

Conclusions

Evidence-based practice is about framing researchable questions as problems arise in clinical practice; searching for the best evidence available to answer those questions; appraising the quality of the evidence available and its applicability to local circumstance; and integrating the external evidence with clinical expertise and patient preferences to improve the quality of care. This introductory chapter has sought to provide insight and guidance into this process. Much fuller accounts are readily available to explore the issues raised in greater depth (Crombie, 1996; Greenhalgh, 1997; Sackett *et al*, 1997).

Key points

* Critical appraisal is a structured way of reading research reports to assess their appropriateness, trustworthiness and implications.

* The first key objective is to check that the right design has been used for the question in hand: cross-sectional blinded comparisons with a gold standard for the assessment of tests; inception cohorts with full follow-up for the elucidation of prognosis; and randomised controlled trials (or systematic reviews of the same) for the assessment of interventions.

* The second objective is to ensure that the study under consideration has been performed to a high standard. Readily available checklists can assist with this assessment of internal validity.

* Deciding whether external evidence applies locally (external validity) involves consideration of differences between the study setting and local circumstances in terms of: the patients seen; the interventions available; the outcomes desired; and the service contexts.

* Evidence alone is insufficient. Evidence needs to be integrated with patients' preferences and values. Such a process utilises clinical expertise and tacit knowledge over explicit checklists.

References

Brennan P, Croft P (1994) Interpreting the results of observational research: chance is not such a fine thing. *Br Med J* **309**: 727–30

Crombie IK (1996) *The Pocket Guide to Critical Appraisal.* BMJ
Publishing, London
Greenhalgh T (1997) *How to Read a Paper: the basics of evidence-based
medicine.* BMJ Publishing, London
Sackett DL, Richardson WS, Rosenberg W, Haynes RB (1997)
Evidence-based Medicine: how to practice and teach EBM. Churchill
Livingstone, London

Section I:
Building blocks

1

Issues in measurement

Huw Davies

Measurement lies at the heart of all quantitative methods in clinical, epidemiological and health services research. If the measures employed lack the essential features of validity and reliability then the conclusions drawn from empirical findings may mislead. Here we explain and explore the desirable features of measurement instruments used in health care research.

Measurement is central to much of health care research. Yet, if the measurement tools used are inadequate then the findings that follow will carry little conviction. Here we explore the desirable features of measurement tools and explain how to assess the suitability of measures used in published studies.

Types of measures

In understanding measurement the first notion to grasp is that different scales can have very different basic properties. At the most basic are **nominal** scales: those that simply define different values that a variable can hold but say nothing about the relationship between those values. For example, a measure of eye colour may simply classify eyes as blue, green, brown etc. With nominal scales it makes no sense to say that one value is more or less than another.

More useful scales (in that they carry more information) are those that are **ordinal**. In ordinal scales, there exists a natural ordering so that it does make sense to say that one value is more or less than another. Examples of such scales would be standard measures of social class or deprivation, measures of educational attainment, and many measures of disease severity. In all these scales there is a natural ordering of values from 'least' to 'most'.

Much of health services research employs such ordinal scales as they are easy to devise and are intuitive in interpretation. However, they are also frequently misused. Although ordinal scales by definition contain a natural ordering, there is nothing in such scales that requires the values to be evenly spaced. For example, if a disease severity measure involved gradings of none, mild, moderate and severe, there is no reason to suppose that 'moderate' lies halfway between 'mild' and 'severe'. This limitation makes it inadmissible to calculate means and standard deviations from ordinal data: medians and inter-quartile ranges are strongly to be preferred. This issue is covered in depth in *Chapter 3*, yet many cases can be found in the literature of the misuse of ordinal scales. For example, when data are presented as 'mean disease severity' or 'mean social class'.

Scales that have true interval properties provide more information about what is measured, and deliver data that can be manipulated statistically. Even here there are pitfalls. Some measures have meaningful intervals but do not have a fixed and independent zero point: this makes calculating ratios problematic. For example, at first sight it might appear that 20 degrees centigrade is twice as hot as 10 degrees. However, the falsity of this becomes clear when we convert to a different scale — fahrenheit. Here 10°C corresponds to 50°F, and 20° C is 68° F. It now appears that 68°F is only 1.36 times as hot as 50°C. This apparent paradox arises because of the essential arbitrariness of the zero in both the fahrenheit and the centigrade scales. When there is no fixed zero we should be careful about inferring that one value is any multiple of another. Such situations might arise for example in many measures of disease severity, physical and psychological functioning, or quality of life.

Measurement properties

Two conceptually distinct but practically intertwined issues bedevil all empirical measures: reliability and validity. **Reliability** relates to the precision of any measuring instrument (and here we are using the term 'instrument' in its broadest sense, encompassing any tool used to measure, including questionnaires). A reliable measure will give the same values on repeated application so long as what is being measured remains unchanged. **Validity**, on the other hand, reflects the extent to which the measures applied are really measuring the desired underlying properties. Clearly then, the properties of reliability and validity are matters of **extent**, rather than being simply present or absent.

Any given measure may be fairly valid but still unreliable. For example, measuring people's height using a simple tape measure may lack precision but still on average be a reasonable estimate of their true height. Conversely, measures may be highly reliable but nonetheless lack validity. For example, measuring height using a wrongly calibrated laser measure may give highly reproducible but nonetheless inaccurate readings.

Ideal measures have a high degree of both reliability and validity, but to some extent there are trade-offs between these: crude measures may sacrifice validity for the sake of reliability.

Exploring reliability

Reliable measures are those that give consistent, precise and repeatable measurements. Clearly this is something that is readily tested empirically, and in that reliability is much easier to establish than validity. One special but important aspect of measurement reliability is that of the consistency within and between raters. Suppose, for example, that clinical measures of disease severity are being estimated by clinicians as part of a research project. Then it is important to know both that each rating clinician is consistent in how s/he grades patients (**intra**-rater reliability) and also that there is consistency between different clinicians (**inter**-rater reliability). These can be tested by getting the same clinician to re-grade a batch of patients seen previously, and by comparing the ratings made by different clinicians on the same group of patients. A high degree of agreement in either case indicates that the measurements used are reliable. However, since a certain amount of agreement is to be expected by chance alone, then this too must be taken into account in any assessment of reliability.

Exploring validity

Validity remains a rather more elusive and somewhat more complicated concept than reliability. Colloquially, validity is concerned with ensuring that we **are** measuring what we **think** we are measuring. Now, when some 'gold-standard' measure exists we can test out validity by comparing the performance of any new measure with that of the gold standard. For example, suppose we wish to develop a simple questionnaire to assess smoking habits, but we know that people are inaccurate reporters of their behaviour in this respect. To assess the validity of our questionnaire, we may try it out on a sample of volunteers and then compare the findings with biochemical measures of cotinine taken from saliva swabs from the same individuals (cotinine is a highly accurate measure of true exposure to tobacco smoke). If the questionnaire findings correlate well with the cotinine levels then this would reassure that the questionnaire is indeed a valid measure of smoking habits.

More often, we do not have a simple readily available gold standard against which to compare any new measuring instrument. That being so, there are several different approaches to establishing the extent of validity. **Face** and **content** validity are terms used to describe whether, on the face of it, the separate items making up a measurement tool seem to cover all the appropriate domains of interest. For example, a measure of physical function designed for assessing elderly patients which did not cover such issues as getting in and out of the bath, or climbing stairs, would be significantly lacking in content validity. **Construct** validity relates to whether or not the measurement tool produces data that are consistent with known patterns. For example, a measure of angina severity should produce data that are consistent with exercise tolerance. Closely related to this is predictive validity — this suggests that the data from a valid measure should be successful in predicting future changes. For example, a disease severity measure that did not correlate with survival would cast doubt on the validity of the instrument used to measure severity. Finally, an important aspect of validity is **sensitivity**: the measures used in any given study should allow us to discriminate between groups in meaningful ways, and should be capable of detecting clinically important changes.

One crucial feature of measures that lack validity is that their deficiencies may vary in systematic ways between groups studied. For example, measuring people's exposure to tobacco smoke is difficult and some deficiencies in validity can be expected. However, the extent of these validity problems may be expected to vary between, for example, healthy people and those recently diagnosed with lung disease. Clearly, such systematic variation may give rise to spurious findings that can mislead.

Assessing the use of measures

In assessing the appropriateness of the measures used in published reports a number of questions are germane. First: what are the scale's basic properties? That is, does the scale have ordinal, interval or ratio properties? If the scale is anything less than a true ratio scale then this limitation will need to be taken into account during analysis and interpretation. Second: is the scale sufficiently reliable, valid and sensitive for the purpose it is being used? Answering this question is not straightforward which then leads us to ask: what efforts have the authors made to test the properties of their measures, and how successful have they been in so doing? Further, because we know that different biases may arise when measures are used with certain groups, we should ask: are there reasons to believe that the reliability/validity will differ systematically between the different study groups? Finally, we need to be aware that measures may perform well in one context (for example, when administered by a professional in a consulting room) but be inadequate in another (for example, when used as part of a self-completed questionnaire). We should also ask: are there contextual issues that may affect the quality of the measures obtained?

Let us now explore just one published example with measurement shortcomings. In 1996, the *Lancet* published a paper examining the use of drink and drugs by university students (Webb *et al*, 1996). The students' consumption was measured by way of a self-completed questionnaire distributed in lectures. There are many ways in which we can speculate that such a measure may mislead. First of all there is the problem of estimating accurately an average level of a highly variable activity. It is likely that respondents' answers will be disproportionately swayed by their most recent experience, so limiting the reliability of the measure.

Validity too will be a problem. For example, those with large consumption of drink and drugs may **under**-report for a variety of reasons, perhaps to do with social desirability. In contrast, some respondents (perhaps through bravado) may report wildly inaccurate **over**-estimates. The crucial point is that we have no way of knowing which of these potential biases will prevail. Further, the context in which the instrument was used (sitting next to one's peers in a crowded lecture theatre at 9.00 am) may well have a marked (but again unpredictable) effect on the responses received. Unfortunately, the only reassurance given by the authors as to the measuring tool's properties was that, 'discussion with students after the questionnaire sessions indicated that their reports were generally accurate'. This seems insufficient to persuade that the measures used would provide a true account of the complex behaviour of students.

In conclusion

Good measurement underlies all the quantitative methods used in health-related research. No matter how good the design, if the measures are flawed then this will always undermine confidence in research findings. Crucially, we can be misled in two ways. The use of imprecise or invalid measures may simply obscure real and important relationships leading us to miss valuable insights. For example, measures that are insensitive to change may miss small but important differences between groups. Perhaps more importantly, the use of flawed measures may purport to reveal features that are in fact only artefacts of the measures used. Measures that are invalid may produce differential responses between groups with different characteristics, leading to erroneous conclusions.

Developing good measures of complex constructs is challenging and arduous. Some helpful texts (Streiner and Norman, 1989; Oppenheim, 1992) provide considerable insights into the process, showing in greater detail how validity and reliability can be established. The complexity and uncertainty of the process is in itself a sound argument for researchers using established instruments wherever possible. At the very least, all published reports should carry a clear statement as to the soundness of the measures used.

Key points

* Good measurement underlies all quantitative research methods.

* Different measures have different scale properties: not all scales have interval or ratio properties.

* Measures should be **reliable**: providing consistent values when the same phenomenon is measured.

* Measures should be **valid**: in essence, capturing the true properties of what is being measured.

* Validity is multi-faceted and complex — both to define and to establish.

* Assessing validity may involve examining the constituent parts of the measure (**content** validity), identifying the consistency of known relationships (**construct** and **predictive** validity); and ensuring that small changes in reality are picked up by changes in the measures recorded (**sensitivity**).

* Validity and reliability may vary depending on the context within which the measures are used.

* Validity and reliability can be explored empirically — and published reports should either use previously validated scales or explain the extent to which validity and reliability have been assessed within the current study.

References

Oppenheim AN (1992) *Questionnaire Design, Interviewing and Attitude Measurement.* Pinter Publishers Ltd, London

Streiner DL, Norman GR (1989) *Health Measurement Scales: a practical guide to their development and use.* Oxford University Press, Oxford

Webb E, Ashton CH, Kelly P, Kamali F (1996) Alcohol and drug use in UK university students. *Lancet* **348**: 922–25

2

Understanding sampling: representativeness matters

Julian Davis, Iain Crombie, Huw Davies

Sampling, or selecting a group of people to represent a whole population, lies at the heart of almost all research designs. There are many ways of going about this, each presenting its own problems. The trick is to obtain a good-sized sample that is truly representative of the population as a whole.

What is sampling?

The use of sampling is seen in many aspects of our daily lives: 'the world's favourite airline', or '8 out of 10 owners said their cats preferred it'. These are statements based upon data collected from a sample of people chosen from the population at large. Sampling will determine what is put on supermarket shelves, or what programme is shown at peak time on TV. These statements do not, of course, actually represent everyone's opinion. They are the result of asking a small number of people and then assuming that what they say will also (broadly) hold true for everyone else.

In medicine, the situation is no different. Research often intends to discover new knowledge about large groups. However, it is usually impractical to conduct studies on all the individuals in these groups. What is commonly done is to select a smaller group of people, the sample, upon whom to conduct the research; and to select the sample in such a way that the results will apply to the larger group of interest. It is in this assumption of generalisability that many of the pitfalls of sampling lie.

Some terminology

Let us pause here briefly to clarify a few terms. First of all, the population is the overall group of people to whom the results of a given piece of research may apply. This is often assumed to mean everyone, but can be much more restricted — think of it as shorthand for 'the population of interest'. For example, a study looking at the usefulness of a new type of foam rubber pad in artificial limbs would not intend to be generalisable to everyone — only to those who actually have artificial limbs. And so the 'population' in this case would be everyone who has an artificial limb. Equally, in examining the effectiveness of a new kidney dialysis fluid, the results would only be intended to be applicable to those patients on dialysis.

Then there is the sample. The sample is a smaller group of people chosen from within the population of interest. They are the ones who will actually take part in the research, and they should have been chosen to be representative of the population as a whole. Sampling is the process of choosing the sample from within the population; and a representative sample is one that is similar in all respects to the target population.

Sampling can allow powerful conclusions to be drawn about the population of interest by collecting data on only a relatively small number of people. Indeed, the data collected from a well-chosen and carefully selected sample can be almost as informative and reliable as that taken from a complete census. All this begs the questions — how should researchers choose who to include and who to reject, and what are the consequences if they get it wrong?

Types of sample, and how to go about obtaining them

Random or probability samples

Random samples (also called probability samples) are the most commonly encountered in medical research, particularly in surveys (Streiner and Norman, 1996). This is because they are generally thought to offer the best approximation to wider populations of interest, and to allow generalisation of the research findings.

A randomly selected sample is one in which the decision about whom to include is left to chance. In the simplest case, you could roll a dice and use the result to decide the fate of each individual: whether to include (say, roll a one) or exclude (roll two-to-six). This would generate a sample on average only one sixth the size of the target population. In practice, probability sampling is usually done using computer-generated numbers. All the possible subjects (the population) are listed, and random numbers used to select the sample. *Box 2.1* (below) shows this in action.

Random numbers can be quirky, however. What this means is that randomness does not always guarantee representativeness, and the sample, once chosen, should be checked to see if it is indeed representative. If not, the researchers should allow for any differences in their analysis.

Even if we accept that probability sampling is the best way to select a sample, there are other stages to sampling that should be reported by researchers. In order to select randomly a group of study subjects, the starting point is a clear definition of the population from which the sample is chosen. The process of deciding who should be in this population is fraught with difficulty, and is the point at which many sampling procedures go awry. To give a simplistic example, if we are attempting to test a new treatment for angina, and we choose to select a sample from those people attending a fitness centre, we are unlikely to include many people who actually suffer from the condition. It matters not how carefully random our sampling is, our sample will not represent the population who may benefit from the new treatment.

Although random sampling can be used for most applications, there are a number of alternative methods. However, these vary both in their complexity and in the degree of bias that may arise. Here are some of the more common variations on the theme, and some of the attractions and pitfalls associated with using them.

Box 2.1: Random selection

❖ Imagine a researcher is selecting a sample of 10 individuals from an electoral register containing 1234 people. The register is listed and numbered from one to 1234. Ten random numbers are generated lying between one and 1234, and these are used to select the corresponding subjects. Thus each person has the same chance of being chosen as the next. This approach is likely to lead to representative samples — more so the larger the sample selected.

For example, we might end up selecting individuals numbered: 4 .... 27 .... 34 .... 154 .... 221 .... 456 ..... 565 .... 768 .... 987 .... and 1232.

Samples of convenience

It may sometimes be expedient to use an easily available population from which to choose samples. This could be, for instance, the patients attending a particular clinic, people registered at a conference, or inmates at a prison. This can simplify the process of obtaining the sample, and if the researcher is actually interested only in the characteristics of individuals in a single setting, then it may be an appropriate method. However, it is more often the case that the resulting sample will not be representative of any particular larger population, and the conclusions that are drawn from the work will not readily be generalisable.

Lack of generalisability is always a problem, but sometimes convenience sampling can provide useful results. An Australian study looking at iron status in city children has shown that sampling children from Childhood Centre registers provided as good a result as random sampling. However, they also found that for a companion survey of lead levels, this method did not work so well (Ranmuthugala *et al,* 1998).

Quota samples

This is the method favoured by market research companies, and can be one way of ensuring that different categories of the population are represented in the sample. The population is categorised, for example, by age, sex, social class, ethnicity etc. Samples are then taken from each of these groupings in proportion to the mix of these factors in the population. That is, if 10% of the population are white males aged 20–40 in social class I, then individuals with these characteristics are selected until this quota of 10% is filled. The serious problem with this approach is that the persons selected within each category may not actually be representative of that category at all. The result is an unpredictable sample composition and consequently unreliable research findings.

Close agreement is possible between random and quota sampling. In Sydney, Australia two surveys were carried out as part of a policy development exercise for health promotion programmes. One used a quota sample of 1700 people, and the other selected a random sample of 480 individuals. There were 15 questions common to the two, and in no case was the result significantly different (Cumming, 1990). Quota sampling may indeed provide acceptable results, but it is often hard to tell from published reports whether it will do so or not.

Cluster sampling

In cluster sampling, the sample is chosen from groups that already exist in some convenient form. An example might be choosing a sample of patients from general practice (Sayer, 1999). A clustering approach would first of all involve selection of a number of specific general practices, followed by selection of patients from within those practices. An important point to note here is that the clusters (in this case, specific general practices) may have very different characteristics, and it is essential to have enough clusters for any important differences to be allowed for. However, so long as a reasonable number of clusters are sampled, this approach can lead to samples that are representative of the target population. The method can also have hidden advantages for the researchers, such as being able to restrict the geographical distribution of a sample to facilitate visits, without compromising the generalisability of the findings.

Stratified sampling

Suppose that we are examining research on possible links between radiation from mobile telephones and skin lesions on the ear. A random sample of those with phones would probably produce more younger and less older people. A stratified sampling technique would first divide the population into age categories, and then sample randomly from within these groups.

In general, if the population being used for a study can easily be divided into groups that differ in terms of the characteristic in which the researchers are interested, then this can be used to improve the precision of any estimates. The population is divided up into groups according to the characteristic in question. Next, a similar fraction is taken from each grouping. This ensures that each group is equally represented in the final sample. However, the selection of individuals from within each group must be random for this system to work.

This method is also suited to populations that are complex in make up. For example, in a population such as Saudi Arabia, which has great social complexity, and many layers of structure, a study of the prevalence of brucellosis required the use of stratified cluster sampling to compensate for the complex nature of societal structure (al-Sekait *et al*, 1992). In reading published research, one should try to assess whether the structure of the population of interest is well suited to a stratified approach.

Sequential or systematic sampling

Population listings may already be organised according to some system that may be helpful to those who keep the records, but not to those who want to select samples. In such circumstances it is not unusual for researchers to select every n^{th} individual, where 'n' is chosen so as to generate a sample of the requisite size. In cases where the original lists are ordered only by name, this systematic approach usually generates a result as good as random sampling (Hagino and Lo, 1998). However, when systematic sampling is used, the reader should be aware that the approach is more prone to bias than simple random sampling.

Qualitative research and purposive sampling

The increased interest in qualitative research methods has also resulted in the wider use of different sampling systems. At a basic level, qualitative research is often concerned with gathering opinions and experiences, and as such it is often appropriate to choose people to take part in a way which makes sure that all groups are included. Although not all qualitative research is done on samples chosen in this way, purposive sampling is an important alternative to more probability based methods (Curtis *et al*, 2000). However, qualitative research does not seek to generalise in the same way as quantitative approaches. Specifically, qualitative research is not concerned with making probabilistic assertions that the patterns seen in the sample will be similar to those seen in the population. Hence assessment of the adequacy of samples used in qualitative research is not based on ideas of representativeness. Instead, different types of generalisability are sought, such as the likely transferability of ideas, theories, understanding and insight from one setting to another (Marshall and Rossman, 1995).

What can go wrong?

We have already mentioned some ways in which a selected sample can end up being unrepresentative of the population from which it comes. There are also ways in which even the best sample may provide unreliable results.

Small sample size

The size of a sample is very important, as all events are subject to the play of chance. A small sample may not show a distribution of characteristics that is all that similar to the target population. To illustrate this, say we randomly select four groups of 20 young people. The first might contain 15 women and 5 men, the second 8 women and 12 men, the third 11 women and 9 men and the fourth 6 women and 14 men. None of the samples is evenly divided between men and women, yet we know that there are roughly equal numbers of men and women in our target population. Because the numbers in the samples were small, none of these samples turned out to be particularly representative. The key point here is that research findings from small samples are uncertain: the larger the sample, the more this uncertainty is reduced.

Unrepresentative populations

If the population from which the sample is selected is itself unrepresentative, the sample will clearly not be any better. For example, suppose a sample is selected at random from a list. If that list is inaccurate, because some people are not on it who should be, or are on it and shouldn't be, the sample will not represent the population. The list may be inaccurate if people have moved away, died, or simply not bothered to register. Importantly, it may be that the very people who do not register are the ones who are of prime interest in the study.

Poor response

Even if the population from which the sample is chosen is accurately described, and the sampling is well carried out, there is still the problem of non-response. Consider a study that involved sending out a questionnaire to a sample of people who had a particular condition. If everyone included in the sample responded to the questionnaire, then the results will reflect accurately the characteristics of the population. However, if the only people who respond are those with, for example, more severe symptoms, or those who live alone, then the results will not reflect the characteristics of the population as a whole.

Misleading conclusions

The inappropriateness of a sampling technique can lead to misleading interpretations of data. For example, random sampling of individuals can lead to underestimates of risk of infection in surveys of sexually transmitted infection (Ghani *et al*, 1998). Here the authors also suggested that allowing for the peculiar nature of sexual partner networks can be achieved by using variants on the theme of cluster sampling.

Summary

In summary, a few simple questions can reveal much about the quality of the sampling in medical research.

How representative is the sample?

It is easy to obtain an unrepresentative sample. What is important when reading and assessing studies is to look to see how hard the researchers tried to make sure their sample was representative. Did they approach the problem systematically? Did they use an appropriate sampling method? Was this rigorously applied, and did they make multiple attempts to contact non-responders?

How good are the data?

It is equally hard to obtain good quality data. How did the researchers go about gathering the data? Did they use previously validated methods (for example questionnaires that had been used in another survey previously)? Did they test their data collection by doing a pilot study (using a smaller sample from an appropriate group)? Were the methods they used sensible (were they trying to use a questionnaire when an interview would have been more appropriate)?

As we have seen, it is the nature of the sample that is the key to the success of much research. Randomised trials, cohort studies, cross-sectional surveys and other study designs all depend upon the appropriateness of their samples for their success. With poor sampling strategies, research findings may prove to be true for the group in which they were determined, but not that generalisable to any wider population of interest.

Key points

* Taking a sample from a population and then drawing conclusions from it is a common feature of most clinical research.

* Samples can be taken using many methods, and it is important to use the right one.

* Each method has its own features, and its own shortcomings.

* Using the wrong method can produce biased and unreliable results.

* The sampling method used should be a factor in the interpretation of research findings.

References

al-Sekait MA, Bamgboye EA, al-Nasser AN (1992) Sampling in epidemiological research: a case study of the prevalence of brucellosis in Saudi Arabia. *J Royal Soc Health* **112**(4): 172–6

Cumming RG (1990) Is probability sampling always better? A comparison of results from a quota and a probability sample survey. *Community Health Stud* **14**(2): 132–7

Curtis S, Gesler W, Smith G (2000) Approaches to sampling and case selection in qualitative research: examples in the geography of health. *Soc Sci Med* **50**(7–8): 1001–14

Ghani AC, Donnelly CA, Garnett GP (1998) Sampling biases and missing data in explorations of sexual partner networks for the spread of sexually transmitted diseases. *Stat Med* **17**(18): 2079–97

Hagino C, Lo RJ (1998) Random *vs* systematic sampling from administrative databases involving human subjects. *J Manipulative Physiol Ther* **21**(7): 454–9

Marshall C, Rossman GB (1995) *Designing Qualitative Research*. Sage, London

Ranmuthugala`G, Karr M, Mira M (1998) Opportunistic sampling from early childhood centres: a substitute for random sampling to determine lead and iron status of pre-school children? *Aust N Z J Public Health* **22**(4): 512–4

Sayer GP (1999) Estimating and generalizing with clustered sampling in general practice. *Aust Fam Physician* **28** Suppl 1: S32–4

Streiner DL, Norman GR (1996) *PDQ Epidemiology*. Mosby, St Louis

3

Informative presentation of summary data

Huw Davies

Many research reports display summary data on study subjects. Seemingly simple tables of data present the mean and standard deviation for each variable. Yet this method of presentation is sometimes less than helpful and at other times it is plain wrong. Ordinal data should not be summarised using means and standard deviations and even interval data are often best not summarised in this way. Medians and percentiles are usually more informative.

Research papers describe research findings. In many papers the first table of data presents a summary description of the research subjects. This is usually so for surveys, cohort studies, case-control studies and clinical trials. More often than not this first table is subtitled 'data are presented as means and standard deviations'. This commonest of headings frequently heralds unhelpful and sometimes misleading data.

Ordinal data

Descriptions of study subjects often include some summary statements on health status. For example, pain severity may be assessed as none, mild, moderate or severe; other symptoms may simply be assessed as present or absent. Numbering health status categories (eg. from none = 0 to severe = 3), or adding up the number of symptoms (from a pre-set list) leads to a handy 'severity score' for each study subject. Sometimes a combination of these approaches is used. For example, to obtain an Apgar score, each of five criteria (heart rate, respiratory effort, muscle tone, response to stimulation and skin colour) are assessed on a scale from nought to two and these numbers are then summed to give a score between nought and ten (Lancet, 1982).

Most areas of health care use simple scoring schemes in this fashion to describe the nature of patients and their problems (Bowling, 1997). These scores vary from subject to subject and provide a useful description of the individuals in the study. But how can these data be combined to indicate both the 'average' value and the amount of variability? Often the response is to quote the mean and the standard deviation (SD). Unfortunately, this is as often inappropriate as it is commonplace.

Data gathered as described above are at best ordinal.[1] That is, we may know the order of different named categories but we do not know anything about the intervals between those categories. For example, we do not know how much worse 'moderate pain' is than 'mild pain', and we have no reason to believe that the difference between mild and moderate pain is the same as that between moderate and severe pain (see *Chapter 1*).

Yet the fact that the categories are conveniently numbered lulls us into believing that these measures have properties that they do not in fact possess (ie. in this case we tend to assume that named points are equidistant). In fact, the numbering is quite arbitrary. For example, numbering pain scores sequentially from 0 to 3 has no more of a basis in reality than (say) assigning scores of none = 0, mild = 5, moderate = 6 and severe = 8. Clearly if we do this then any calculated means and standard deviations will also change.

The example in *Table 3.1* shows that as the scoring scheme is altered the group mean varies from less than mild pain (scoring scheme B) to more than moderate pain (scoring scheme C). This summary measure is, therefore, not a helpful descriptor of the group as a whole as it is so dependent on the (arbitrary) scoring scheme chosen. The same arguments apply to the calculation of the standard deviation from ordinal data: SDs calculated from ordinal data are inadmissible.

Non-normality

Even when the measures used have meaningful intervals (eg. age, weight, drug consumption, number of days spent in hospital), the mean and the standard deviation may not always be the best way of describing the data. The values from every subject are used to

---

1   And they may not even be ordinal if diverse categories are being summed. For example, if three symptoms are scored 0 (absent) or 1 (present) then the resulting 'severity' score will not be ordinal if one symptom is more serious an indicator than the other two put together. But that is another story.

Description	Number of subjects	Scoring scheme used (score allocated to each pain category)		
		A	B	C
None	15	0	0	1
Mild	22	1	5	3
Moderate	18	2	6	10
Severe	16	3	8	30
Mean score		1.5	4.9	11.1
SD		1.1	2.8	11.1

Table 3.1: Effect of various scoring schemes on the mean and SD

calculate the mean and this can sometimes mean that the mean is not all that typical of the group. For example, if nine people each spend less than a week in hospital and the tenth person spends six months, then the mean length of stay will be about three weeks. This does not reflect any member of the group's experience and it is therefore not a particularly informative summary measure. The mean may be disproportionately influenced by a few extreme values and can be misleading.

The standard deviation (SD) likewise may not always be all that helpful. The SD describes the amount of 'spread' or variation in the data. It is most useful when the data are symmetrical and roughly normal (Altman and Bland, 1995). If these conditions hold, then about two-thirds of any given sample will lie between the mean minus one SD and the mean plus one SD (and around 95% will lie in the range mean ± two SDs). These rules of thumb give the reader a quick and easy feel for the study group.

Unfortunately, if the data are skewed (ie. not symmetric at all but with the data spread out more on one side than the other) these ready ranges using the SD are not helpful: the rules of thumb no longer apply. Health data are frequently skewed. For example, although most people will be discharged quickly some will stay as inpatients for long periods; although most people will need modest amounts of pain relieving drugs, some patients will require much larger doses. The problem is that many reports simply tell us the means and SDs but do not indicate anything further — leaving us to guess whether the mean ± two SDs is meaningful. Sometimes we can tell that it is not (Altman and Bland, 1996). In extreme cases, creating a range of ± two SDs can lead to nonsense, for example, patients with apparently negative drug consumption (Rosenberg *et al*, 1996) (is this drug production?); or negative anxiety, depression and co-morbidity (Grubb *et al*, 1996) (lucky people).

Sometimes the errors are compounded with means and SDs quoted for ordinal data (Kanakoudis *et al*, 1996). Applying the rule (mean ± 2 SDs) to the data in *Table 3.1* (schemes B and C) leads to the expectation that a fair few of the study group have less than no pain (pleasure perhaps?).

Percentiles

If the SD does not convey meaningful information then why quote it? The pitfalls described can readily be avoided by using percentiles instead of the mean and the SD. Percentiles are a way of dividing the study subjects into different groups depending on the value of a particular variable (Altman and Bland, 1994). For example, the 50th percentile for (say) height is the value such that half the group are taller and half are shorter. The 50th percentile is usually known as the median. It is another sort of average and is often more useful than the more usual arithmetic mean.

Percentiles are easy to grasp and highly versatile. For example, the interval from the 25th percentile to the 75th percentile (called the interquartile range) defines half of the study group. If we calculate the interquartile range for height then a quarter of the group will be shorter than the lower value, half of the group will lie within the range, and the final quarter will be taller than the upper value. Simple and easy to visualise. Other ranges may be similarly useful: for example, the interval from the 5th percentile to the 95th percentile includes fully 90% of the subjects; and in the extreme the full range (nought percentile to 100 percentile) includes everyone. Which intervals are displayed will depend on the purpose (for example, to describe the main group or indicate the extent of the unusual). Whichever intervals are presented they at least have the merit of being immediately interpretable.

Percentiles can also be used for ordinal data. Here it is better to let the categories define the percentiles displayed rather than to try to force the data into fixed percentile ranges. For example, one could present the range for patients with mild to moderate pain (in the case of the data in *Table 3.1*, 22% –77%) thus indicating that 22% had less than mild pain and 23% had more than moderate pain. Similarly, for Apgar scores, one could indicate the proportion of babies scoring less than 5, or the proportion scoring between 6 and 9 inclusive. Data presentation in this form requires no distributional assumptions and is immediately informative rather than potentially misleading.

Concluding remarks

The nature of research is such that study subjects and their outcomes are frequently described using ordinal data (eg. pain scores, sedation scores, disease severity). Even when the measurements used are continuous on interval or ratio scales, the data obtained are often highly skewed (eg. time to recovery, time to discharge, drug consumption). Using means and standard deviations in these cases is unhelpful, sometimes misleading and needless.

These problems are common, occurring in almost every issue of some journals. Once sensitised, readers will scarcely be able to avoid noticing inappropriate means and standard deviations in published reports. Yet simple solutions exist which are readily implemented using modern statistical packages. Instead of routinely using means and standard deviations, authors should ask themselves the following two questions:

- are these interval data?
- are these data roughly normal?

If the answer to either question is 'no' then medians and other percentiles may be a more honest and a more helpful way of presenting the data.

Key points

* Ordinal data (ie. those relating to ordered categories such as 'mild', 'moderate' and 'severe') should not be summarised using means or standard deviations. Reports which present data in this way are suspect.

* Ordinal data are best described using percentiles.

* Even interval data (ie. continuous measurements such as time to recovery, length of stay etc) may not be best summarised using means and standard deviations.

* If the data are not roughly normal in distribution then percentiles should be used in preference to means and standard deviations.

* If the mean value plus or minus two standard deviations leads to nonsense (eg. meaningless negative values) then the data are poorly presented and may mislead.

References

Altman DG, Bland JM (1994) Quartiles, quintiles, centiles, and other quantiles. *Br Med J* **309**: 996

Altman DG, Bland JM (1995) The normal distribution. *Br Med J* **310**: 298

Altman DG, Bland JM (1996) Detecting skewness from summary data. *Br Med J* **313**: 1200

Anonymous (1982) The value of the Apgar score. *Lancet*, 19 June: 1393–4

Bowling A (1997) *Measuring Health. A Review of Quality of Life Measurement Scales*. Open University Press, Milton Keynes

Grubb NR, O'Carroll R, Cobbe SM, Sirel J, Fox KAA (1996) Chronic memory impairment after cardiac arrest outside hospital. *Br Med J* **313**: 143–6

Kanakoudis F, Petrou A, Michaloudis D, Chortaria G, Konstantinidou A (1996) Anaesthesia for intra-peritoneal perfusion of hyperthermic chemotherapy. *Anaesthesia* **51**(11): 1033–36

Rosenberg J, Overgaard H, Anderson M, Rasmussen V, Schulze S (1996) Double blind randomised controlled trial of effect of metoprolol on myocardial ischaemia during endoscopic cholangiopancreatography. *Br Med J* **313**: 258–61

4

Describing and estimating: use and abuse of SD and SE

Huw Davies

Summarising data using means and standard deviations (SDs) is commonplace in research reports. Many papers also present means and standard errors (SEs). But when should the standard deviation be used and when is the standard error appropriate? Published reports are frequently confusing and inconsistent in their use of SDs and SEs. This chapter clarifies the meaning and appropriate roles for these two important measures. The standard deviation is used when describing study subjects and the standard error is used when estimating the precision with which findings from the study sample can be extrapolated to other groups.

One of the commonest rubrics in research reports is 'data are presented as means and standard deviations'. The mean tells us something about the average subject and the standard deviation conveys information on how individual subjects differ from this average (ie. the standard deviation tells of the amount of variability in the data). *Chapter 3* described some of the errors that can be hidden by such a seemingly simple statement.

Sometimes, however, the rubric reads, 'data are presented as means and standard errors'. Why the difference? When should the standard deviation (SD) be used and when is the standard error (SE) appropriate? Here we seek to clarify the different roles of the SD and the SE to aid both reader and writer alike.

Presenting research data

Presentation of data in research reports is often in two parts. First the study subjects are described and then the findings are interpreted to assess their wider implications. In good papers these stages are clearly separated but in some reports the distinction between them is unclear. Yet knowing whether you are simply describing or whether you are extrapolating from these descriptions is crucial if the appropriate statistical approaches are to be used.

Describing the study subjects

Early in any research report the study subjects will be (or should be) described. This description will usually clarify at least two features: the nature of the average subject and the extent of variability between the subjects. The average is usually expressed using the arithmetic mean, the median or sometimes the mode. It tells us, for example, whether study subjects are (on average) old or young, heavy or light, tall or short.

Spread

The average provides a convenient summary of the data but tells us nothing about how individuals differ from one another. For example, if the mean age is 50 we may want to know whether the subjects are all middle aged (low variability), or whether substantial numbers are very young or very old (high variability). Different measures of variability are: the range (difference between the smallest and the largest value), the interquartile range (a range which captures the middle half of the study subjects [Altman and Bland, 1994]) and the standard deviation.

Calculating the standard deviation

The standard deviation (SD) is usually given as a formula (*Box 4.1*). However, it makes more sense to think first what the SD is trying to express. The SD measures the spread of the data — like the range does. But unlike the range (which just uses the highest and lowest values), the SD uses every data point. It is calculated by first measuring the distance of every subject from the mean value $(X-x_i)$. Because these values will sometimes be positive (when the subject value is less than the mean) and sometimes be negative (when the subject value is more than the mean), each of these distances is squared. Now we can work out the average of this squared distance by adding them up and dividing by the number of study subjects.[1] Finally, because we squared the distances in the first place, taking the square root now means the SD can be expressed in the original units. Thus the SD is simply a measure of the 'average distance' between the mean and each of the subject values.

Box 4.1: Formula for SD of a sample mean

$$SD = \sqrt{\frac{\sum (X-x_i)^2}{n-1}}$$

In this formula X is the mean value, and x_i is each of the individual values in turn. The sigma sign ($\sum$) simply means 'calculate the sum of $(X-x_i)^2$ for each of the individual values x_i'. The size of the sample is n.

Interpreting the SD

Interpreting the SD is relatively straightforward. A large SD means lots of variability in the data; ie. many study subjects who are greatly different from the mean value. A small SD tells us the opposite: few study subjects are greatly different from the average. To make these statements more precise we would need to know more about the individual values and the shape of the distribution. Fortunately, many data sets have a distinctive shape which is symmetrical and roughly normal (this does not mean 'usual' but is another name for the Gaussian distribution [Altman and Bland, 1995]). If this is so, a simple rule of thumb can be applied to the data which greatly extends the usefulness of the SD: about two-thirds of any given sample will lie between the mean minus one SD and the mean plus one SD (and around 95% will lie in the range mean ± two SDs).

Thus knowing the mean and SD, and (better still) knowing that the distribution is roughly normal, gives us a clear picture of the study subjects. But that is all the sample SD tells us: it simply describes the variability in the study subjects and says nothing about any wider group about whom we may be interested.

---

1 In practice, when calculating the SD of a sample, we divide by one less than the sample size. This gives a slight technical advantage (it means the SD is an unbiased estimator of the real population variance) but it makes little difference to the values obtained. For samples greater than 10 the difference is less than 10%, for samples greater than 100 the difference is less than 1%.

Making inferences from the study subjects

Detailed descriptions are all very well, but any single study group is only of so much interest. Research is about generating new and useful knowledge which is **generalisable**. Therefore a key concern is what the findings on any particular group can tell us about others who were not included in the study sample. Patients elsewhere for example, or future patients perhaps. We are interested in making inferences from our sample to a wider group of interest. It is in making inferences that the standard error (SE) becomes an appropriate tool.

If the study sample is similar to the wider group of interest then the findings from the study sample will reflect the features of this wider group.[2] Intuitively, it makes sense that if the sample is very small (not much information) or if the study subjects are highly variable (much uncertainty), then our estimates of the nature of the wider group of interest are also likely to be more uncertain. The standard error (SE) helps us determine how precisely the sample findings are likely to reflect the larger group.

Why 'error'?

The standard error is confusingly named. It is not about errors as in mistakes. In essence it tells us how far in error our sample values are likely to be when used to estimate the (unknown) features of the wider group of interest.

Defining the SE

The SE is in fact the standard deviation of a very special distribution. Consider the mean value of some variable in a study sample, say height. Suppose a different (random) sample had been taken — then the mean value for height obtained would be likely to be slightly

---

2   This is a very big IF. Ideally, the sample will have been drawn randomly from the wider group of interest such that each member of the wider group had an equal chance of being included in the sample. In practice this is rarely attained, not least because the wider group of interest may encompass future patients (for example) who clearly have no chance of being included in the current sample. Nevertheless, due consideration of the reasonableness of this assumption should be made before inferences are made (see Brennan and Croft, 1994 and *Chapter 2*).

different. Now, suppose numerous different samples were taken (all the same size and all drawn in the same way). Lots of different mean heights would be obtained, some smaller and some larger than our original. The standard error is simply the standard deviation of these different mean values (and the distribution of these mean values is called the sampling distribution of the mean).

Of course, in practice, we almost never do take repeated samples like this. Fortunately, the standard error can be calculated from the sample data. The SE of any mean calculated on a random sample is simply the standard deviation divided by the square root of the number of study subjects in the sample.

Using the SE

Knowing the SE of a sample mean enables us to say something about the likely real mean of the wider group of interest. Calculating an interval using the sample mean ± 2 SEs creates an interval which most of the time encloses the true mean (about 95% for samples of a reasonable size — say >30). Thus the role of the standard error is not in describing the sample at all, but in **estimating** the precision with which findings from the sample estimate the real (and unknown) values in the wider group of interest.

Conclusion

Even a cursory glance at the literature reveals some confusion over the appropriate use of standard deviations and standard errors. Tables presenting simple descriptive data frequently make erroneous use of the SE, even in reputable journals. Perhaps because the SE is always considerably smaller than the SD authors think that using it in preference will lend (albeit spurious) precision to their data.

Whatever the reason for the confusion it is unfortunate and easily avoidable. The SD allows the reader of a research report to grasp the nature of the study subjects, for instance, assessing whether the study subjects are similar to local groups. The SE in turn allows the reader to understand how precisely the findings from the sample are likely to estimate the characteristics of the wider group from which the sample was drawn (once bias has been taken into account [Brennan and Croft, 1994]). SDs describe the data and SEs estimate population parameters using the data. D for describing and E for estimating. Different measures for different jobs.

Key points

* The standard deviation (SD) is a description of the variability in a sample.

* The standard error (SE) is a measure of the precision with which a mean from the sample estimates the mean in some wider group of interest.

* Therefore the SD is used for **describing** and the SE is used for **estimating**.

* SEs can only be interpreted once the representativeness of the sample has been considered.

References

Altman DG, Bland JM (1994) Quartiles, quintiles, centiles, and other quantiles. *Br Med J* **309**: 996

Altman DG, Bland JM (1995) The normal distribution. *Br Med J* **310**: 298

Brennan P, Croft P (1994) Interpreting the results of observational research: chance is not such a fine thing. *Br Med J* **309**: 727–30

5

Interpreting measures of effect

Huw Davies

A confusing number of measures are used to describe the effect sizes from clinical trials or systematic reviews. Absolute measures (such as the absolute risk reduction or the number needed to treat) and relative measures (such as the relative risk reduction, the relative risk or the odds ratio) may give not just different numerical answers but convey different messages. This chapter describes the role and meaning of the different measures and advises on their interpretation. A key message is the importance of taking into account the initial risk when assessing effect sizes from published studies.

Evidence-based medicine (EBM) requires that all doctors read and appraise evidence of clinical effectiveness. Not only must doctors be able to assess the quality of a trial or systematic review, they must also be able to understand and interpret the measures used to describe the size of any therapeutic effects. This may not be straightforward.

There is a confusing range of ways in which any therapeutic effects seen in clinical trials can be described (*Table 5.1*). Yet the way information is presented can have an impact on our response to that information. For example, when presented with data on the impact of a cardiac rehabilitation programme, health purchasers showed strong support for the programme when the size of effect was described as 'reducing the rate of deaths by 20%'. However, when the programme was described as 'increasing patient survival from 84% to 87%' they were much less impressed (Fahey *et al*, 1995). In fact, these two statements are equivalent.

Users of information on treatment effects should have a clear understanding of the meaning of the different measures and be aware of the pitfalls in their interpretation. The ability to convert between the measures may also assist when assessing information from different published sources.

Table 5.1: Summary of effect measures

Measure of effect	Abbrev	Description	No effect	Total success
Relative risk	RR	Risk of death[1] in the treated group divided by the risk of death in the untreated group. Usually expressed as a decimal proportion.	RR=1	RR=0
Odds ratio	OR	Odds of death in the treated group divided by the odds of death in the untreated group. Usually expressed as a decimal proportion.	OR=1	OR=0
Relative risk reduction	RRR	Proportion of the risk of death removed by treatment. Usually expressed as a percentage.	RRR=0%	RRR=100%
Absolute risk reduction	ARR	Absolute change in risk; risk of death in the untreated minus the risk of death in the treated group. Usually expressed as a percentage.	ARR=0%	ARR=initial risk (%)
Number needed to treat	NNT	Number of patients who need to be treated to prevent one death. This is the reciprocal of the absolute risk reduction.[2]	NNT=∞	NNT=1/initial risk

1: Although 'death' is used in each of these examples, any other 'event' could be tracked in a similar way.

2: The NNT is the reciprocal of the ARR expressed as a decimal fraction, not the reciprocal of the ARR expressed as a percentage.

First things first

In some areas evidence on effectiveness has been nicely summarised by the Cochrane Collaboration or the NHS Centre for Reviews and Dissemination (NHS CRD). This makes appraisal easier as readers of the output from these reputable sources can be reasonably confident that the evidence has been collated in a rigorous and meticulous manner, and so are able to concentrate more on assessing the meaning of the findings in their own local context.

However, evidence from less rigorous sources (that is, almost everywhere else) requires a more careful assessment of its trustworthiness. Single studies, in particular, always require a more-or-less forensic assessment of study design and execution before interpretation of the findings.

Presence of bias

Studies of the benefits (or otherwise) of health care interventions can be flawed (biased) in myriad different ways. If a study is seriously flawed, confidence in the meaning of the findings is undermined. There are many useful guides to study quality available (Crombie, 1996; Guyatt *et al*, 1993; Guyatt *et al*, 1994; Sackett *et al*, 1997; see also *Chapters 14* and *15*). In essence, EBM practitioners are looking for prospective studies with randomised controls; full follow-up of all patients; and blinding of both patients and health care professionals. Any analysis should check that the groups were equivalent at the start and should compare groups on the basis of their initial allocation to treatment group or control (an intention-to-treat analysis). These bare bones outline the requirements of good studies which may lead to trustworthy findings. However, as always, the devil is in the detail. It is no simple matter to detect not just the presence of bias but to assess its likely impact and the extent to which it might undermine or even vitiate the study findings. Yet this critique of study design, execution and analysis must be done before gauging the size of any therapeutic effect (Brennan and Croft, 1994).

Measures of effect

The key measures of effect size are described below (and summarised in *Table 5.1*). The focus is on assessing differences between treated and control groups in their rates of certain dichotomous events. These events may either be bad things (eg. death, stroke, asthma attack, hospital admission) which treatment is intended to prevent; or good things (eg. recovery, ulcer healing, 50% reduction in pain, discharge to community) which treatment is intended to promote.

Absolutes and relatives

Consider survival after a myocardial infarction. Suppose 25% of patients in the control group die within one month, and only 20% of those in the treated group (say a new clot-buster) die. A difference of 5%. If the study was well conducted then our estimate of the impact of treatment is that it saves an additional 5% of those treated. This 5% is called the **absolute risk reduction**.

Alternatively, we could ask what proportion of deaths are prevented? In this case the 5% absolute reduction is 20% of the death rate seen in the control group. This 20% reduction in the death rate is the **relative risk reduction**.

Another way of looking at this is to say that the risk of dying in the treated group is only 80% of the risk of dying in the control group (because 20% is 80% of 25%). This is termed the **relative risk**. Unsurprisingly, the relative risk plus the relative risk reduction always add to 100%.

The **absolute** risk reduction examines the number of events prevented by treatment as a proportion of all patients treated. The **relative** risk reduction looks at the number of events prevented as a proportion of the number of events expected. Hence absolute measures look at the overall picture, whereas relative measures emphasise benefits (eg. lives saved) but ignore wasted effort (eg. patients treated who would have survived anyway).

Absolute and relative measures are both fair and reasonable ways of presenting data — so long as there is no confusion as to which is being examined at any one time. Relative risk reductions are always bigger than the absolute risk reductions, more so as the initial risk rate gets smaller (*Table 5.2*). That is why relative risk reductions (or just the relative risks themselves) can often look impressive even when the absolute changes are small.

Table 5.2: Absolute risk reduction for a given initial risk and relative risk reduction

Initial risk	Relative risk reduction		
	10%	20%	50%
50%	5%	10%	25%
20%	2%	4%	10%
10%	1%	2%	5%
5%	0.5%	1%	2.5%
1%	0.1%	0.2%	0.5%

Interpreting both absolute and relative measures should be carried out in the light of the initial risk rates. When only one measure is given it is worthwhile calculating the other and asking:

- what proportion of patients treated will gain any additional benefit (the absolute impact)?

- what proportion of the problem is removed (the relative impact)?

Odds ratios

Sometimes papers present odds ratios rather than relative risks.[1] In almost all cases likely to be encountered the odds ratio can be interpreted as though it were a relative risk (Davies *et al*, 1998). A word of caution though: the odds ratio will always overstate the case. When the odds ratio is less than one it will be smaller than the actual relative risk, and when the odds ratio is greater than one it will be larger than the relative risk. However, the discrepancy only becomes significant when the effect sizes are large and qualitative judgements are unlikely to be unsettled by any discrepancy. A fuller description of odds, odds ratios and how to interpret them is given in Davies, 1998 and in a past edition of *Bandolier* (Deeks, 1996).

Number needed to treat

More recently a new and useful measure has appeared on the scene and received widespread approval. The number needed to treat (NNT) is a measure of how many patients must be treated to get one good event (or prevent one bad one). For example, how many patients (on average) must be given thrombolysis to prevent one death at 30 days? This is the NNT.

In the example used earlier, mortality after myocardial infarction was reduced from 25% in the control group to 20% in the treated group. That is, for every 100 patients treated, 20 die anyway, 75 would have lived regardless and five are saved by treatment (assuming an unbiased study). Therefore twenty patients must be treated to prevent one death: the NNT is 20. In practice, calculation of the NNT is simple: it is just the reciprocal of the absolute risk reduction.

1   The concept of odds is often confusing to people used to thinking of risks. Risk is calculated by dividing the number of events (say death) by the total number at risk of that event. It is the proportion of people who suffer any given event. Odds however are calculated by dividing the number of those with an event by the numbers **not** having that event. Thus, if the risk of dying is p (as a proportion) then the odds of dying are simply $p/(1-p)$. That is, the odds is the ratio of dying to not dying. The odds ratio is simply the ratio of the odds of death (or whatever) between the treated and the control group.

The NNT naturally incorporates the underlying risk (applying as it does to defined groups) and is readily understood by doctors and many patients. For this reason and others (it can be adjusted for patients at different baseline risks) the NNT has rapidly gained popularity (Cook and Sackett, 1995).

NNTs have great intuitive appeal but they are not without drawbacks. Because they incorporate the underlying risk, they are only applicable to groups of patients with a similar underlying risk. For example, if an NNT has been calculated from a study of patients with high risk it will not be applicable to patient groups with low risk. Further, the lower the NNT the more effective the therapy, but even totally effective therapies may have quite high NNTs. This is because the lowest value the NNT can take is the reciprocal of the initial risk. If the initial risk of an event is 10% then even a treatment that is totally effective in removing all this risk will have an NNT of 10. NNTs for low risk groups may look unimpressively high even when the intervention is highly effective.

Play of chance

Having a high quality unbiased study and clearly described effect sizes is not enough to finish the job. Doubts remain as to whether we are being led astray by chance. If an effect is found could it just be due to random fluctuations? If so, then confidence in the therapeutic effect of the intervention would be misplaced. If no effect is seen, could this also be due to chance and might therapeutic opportunities be being missed? Answering these questions is the role of p-values and confidence intervals which are examined in *Chapter 6*.

Conclusions

Treatment effect sizes can be displayed in different ways which either emphasise or underplay the benefits. Relative measures focus on benefits whereas absolute measures look at the whole picture. Using both and interpreting them in the light of the initial risk rate can give a more balanced view of the effect size.

The NNT highlights the number of patients treated without benefit in the pursuit of one therapeutic success. It gives a readily understandable measure which incorporates the underlying risk. However, the NNT is specific to groups of patients with a given underlying risk and generalisation to other groups requires care.

Key points

* The ways in which treatment effect sizes are described can influence our response to the findings from clinical trials and systematic reviews.

* Using the absolute risk reduction gives a picture of the overall benefits achieved from all patients treated.

* Using the relative risk or relative risk reduction emphasises the benefits while ignoring patients who gain no benefit.

* Small absolute risk reductions may reflect large relative risk reductions when the initial risk is low.

* The NNT is a convenient and readily understandable measure of effect that incorporates the effects of the underlying risk.

* NNTs are specific to groups with the same initial risk and therefore they should not be generalised without adjustment to other groups at higher or lower risk.

References

Brennan P, Croft P (1994) Interpreting the results of observational research: chance is not such a fine thing. *Br Med J* **309**: 727–30

Cook RJ, Sackett DL (1995) The number needed to treat: a clinically useful measure of treatment effect. *Br Med J* **310**: 452–4

Crombie IK (1996) *The Pocket Guide to Critical Appraisal*. BMJ Publishing, London

Davies HTO, Crombie IK, Tavakoli M (1998) When can odds ratios mislead? *Br Med J* **314**: 689–91

Deeks J (1996) Swots corner: what is an odds ratio? *Bandolier* **3**(3): 6–7

Fahey T, Griffiths S, Peters TJ (1995) Evidence-based purchasing: understanding results of clinical trials and systematic reviews. *Br Med J* **311**: 1056–60

Guyatt GH, Sackett DL, Cook DJ (1993) Users' guides to the medical literature. II. How to use an article about therapy or prevention. A. Are the results of the study valid? *JAMA* **270**(21): 2598–601

Guyatt GH, Sackett DL, Cook DJ (1994) Users' guides to the medical literature. II. How to use an article about therapy or prevention. B. What were the results and will they help me in caring for my patients? *JAMA* **271**(1): 59–63

Sackett DL, Richardson WS, Rosenberg W, Haynes RB (1997) *Evidence-based Medicine: how to practice and teach EBM*. Churchill Livingstone, London

6

Assessing chance variability in comparisons

Huw Davies

Chance variability can obscure the nature of the world and this is a particular problem in assessing the findings from clinical trials. P-values and confidence intervals provide a guide to the play of chance but are easily misinterpreted. There are two basic ways in which we can be misled. Firstly, by assuming that 'statistical significance' means that the study demonstrates a real and important effect; and secondly, by assuming that 'non significance' demonstrates that there is in reality no effect. Neither of these assumptions is true. This chapter explains the correct interpretation of both p-values and confidence intervals when used to assess the findings from clinical trials.

Clinical trials aim to generate new knowledge on the effectiveness (or otherwise) of health care interventions. However, as trials are carried out on only a sample of patients this raises a dilemma: are the findings discovered about the sample also likely to be true about other similar groups of patients? Before we can answer such a question two issues need to be addressed. Does any apparent treatment benefit arise because of the way the study has been conducted (bias) or could it arise simply because of chance? Here we cover only briefly the importance of assessing bias but focus more on assessing the play of chance. Common pitfalls in the interpretation of p-values and confidence intervals are described and advice is given on avoiding them.

Bias

Bias is a term that covers any systematic errors in the way the study was designed, executed or interpreted. Common failures in trials are lack of (or failure in) randomisation (leading to unbalanced groups); poor blinding (leading to unfair treatment and biased assessments) and losses to follow-up. Assessment in these areas is crucial before the results from any trial can be assessed and many useful guides exist to assist this process (Crombie, 1996; see also *Chapters 14* and *15*). Interpretation of the effects of chance are only meaningful once bias has been excluded as an explanation for any observed difference (Brennan and Croft, 1994).

Chance variability

Two main approaches are used in assessing the play of chance: the ubiquitous p-value and, growing in prominence in more recent years, the confidence interval. Although they might appear dissimilar, the theory and calculations underlying these two approaches are largely the same.

P-values

The logic of p-values is convoluted. Suppose a new treatment appears to outperform the standard therapy in a research study. We are interested in assessing whether this apparent effect is likely to be real or could just be a chance finding.

In calculating the p-value we **suppose** that there really is no true difference between the two treatments.[1] We then calculate how likely we are to see the difference that we have observed just by chance if our supposition is true (ie. if there really is no true difference). This is the p-value.

So: the p-value is the probability that we would observe effects as big as those seen in the study if there was really no difference between the treatments. If p is small, then the findings are unlikely to have arisen by chance, and we reject the idea that there is no difference between the two treatments. If p is large, the observed difference is plausibly a chance finding, and we do not reject the idea that there is no difference between the treatments. Note that we do not reject the idea, but we do not accept it either: we are simply unable to say one way or another until other factors have been considered (see 'Powerful studies', *p. 44*).

Although they are often confused as such, the p-value is **not** the probability that the observed difference is real. The probability

---

1   For the technically minded, this supposition is called 'the null hypothesis'.

relates not to the chances of there being a real effect — but to the chances of these data being found if there was no real difference.

But what do we mean by a 'small' p-value (one small enough to cause us to reject the idea that there was really no difference)? By convention, p-values of less than 0.05 are considered 'small'. That is, if p is less than 0.05 then there is a less than one-in-twenty chance that a difference as big as that seen in the study could have arisen by chance if there was really no true difference. With p-values this small (or smaller) we say that the results from the trial are statistically significant (unlikely to have arisen by chance). Smaller p-values (say $p<0.01$) are sometimes called 'highly significant' because they indicate that the observed difference would happen less than one-time-in-a-hundred if there was really no true difference.

Getting it wrong: finding things which are not there

There are several ways in which we can come to erroneous conclusions after examining a p-value. First, if the p-value is small (less than 0.05) we will note that the observed difference is unlikely to have arisen by chance. We usually conclude that there is a difference between the two treatments. However, just because an event is unlikely does not mean that it will not happen. By definition, about one-in-twenty significant p-values will be spurious — arising simply from chance. We may be misled by chance into believing in something which is not real.[2]

It is a frustrating but unavoidable feature of p-values that around one-in-twenty will mislead — but we do not know which of any given set of p-values is doing the misleading. This observation cautions against generating too many p-values: the more p-values calculated in any given study the greater the chance that at least some of them will be spurious. Thus, clinical trials which show significance in only one or two subgroups are unconvincing — such significance may be deceptive. Unless specific subgroup analyses have been specified in advance, p-values calculated for any difference other than the primary endpoint for the whole group should be eyed with suspicion.

---

2   Technically, this is a Type I error.

Statistical significance and clinical significance

Statistical significance is also sometimes misinterpreted as signifying an important result. Yet significance testing simply asks whether the data produced in a study are compatible with the notion of no difference between the new and control interventions. Rejecting equivalence of the two interventions does not necessarily mean that we accept there is an **important** difference between them. A large study may identify as statistically significant a fairly small difference. It is then quite a separate judgement to assess the clinical significance of this difference. In assessing the importance of significant results it is the size of the effect not just the size of the significance that matters.

Getting it wrong again: failing to find things which are there

A further error that we may make is to conclude from a large p-value (greater than 0.05) that there is no effect, when in fact there is.[3] Equating non-significance with 'no effect' is a frequent and damaging misconception. A non-significant p-value simply tells us that the observed difference is consistent with there being no difference between the two groups. We are unable to reject this possibility of no difference. However, in many cases the observed difference will also be compatible with a range of effect sizes which are important, and thus we are unable to reject these possibilities either. Just because we have not found a treatment effect does not mean that there is no treatment effect (Altman and Bland, 1995). The crucial question is how hard have we looked?

Powerful studies

In clinical trials, how much effort has been spent looking is called the 'power' of a study. The power is the chances of a study finding effects of a given size if they are really present. It is largely a function of the sample size.[4] Well-written study reports usually contain an estimate of the power of the reported study. Regrettably, many reports do not provide these details.

Small studies have low power to detect even large and worth-

3   Technically, this is a Type II error.
4   Power is also a function of the variability of the outcome being measured, the significance cut-off being used (termed 'alpha') and the minimally important difference being looked for (Florey, 1993).

while treatment effects. A non-significant result in a small study provides little real information: there may be no true effect but, on the other hand, there could be a large and important true effect which is simply obscured by the chance variability inherent in small numbers. In contrast, a non-significant finding from a large study can be genuinely useful as it may exclude the possibility of anything other than small effects.

The difficulty of establishing safety

Clinical trials do not just report on effectiveness — many also comment on the apparent safety of the treatment under test. A common assumption is that if no deleterious side-effects are observed then the new therapy is safe: an erroneous assumption. A useful statistical approximation is that if no events are reported then the true underlying rate of those events is unlikely to be higher than 300 divided by the sample size (Eypasch *et al*, 1995). No deaths reported from a study of size 100 means that the true underlying death rate may be as high as 3% and the zero deaths observed was just fortuitous. Of course, the true death rate could also be zero. The point is, that even studies of several hundred patients are unable to exclude the possibility of small rates of damaging side-effects (that is, they have low power to detect them).

False dichotomies

The problem with p-values is that they only give us one piece of information: whether or not we should reject the idea that there is no difference between the two treatments. If we do not reject the possibility that the treatments are the same we are no clearer as to how they may actually differ.

Further, a dichotomous choice between 'reject' and 'not reject' may not always be helpful. For example, a p-value of 0.045 may arise from an almost identical set of data as one which produces a p-value of 0.055. Yet the decision rule of statistical significance pushes us into interpreting these two (very similar) sets of results in rather different ways (significant in one case, non-significant in the other). Fortunately confidence intervals overcome some of the difficulties intrinsic to p-values (Gardner and Altman, 1986).

Confidence intervals

Confidence intervals (CIs) take as their starting point the results from the study. The question they then answer is 'what is the range of real effects that are compatible with these data?'. The confidence interval is a range about the main measure of effect (relative risk reduction, absolute risk reduction, NNT or whatever, see *Chapter 5*) which 95% of the time will contain the true value.

This allows us to do two things. First, if the CI embraces the value of no effect (eg. no difference between two treatments as shown by a relative risk equal to one or an absolute difference equal to zero, *Chapter 5*) then the findings are non-significant. If the CI does not embrace the value of no difference then the findings are statistically significant. Thus confidence intervals provide the same information as a p-value. But more than this. The upper and lower extremities of the confidence interval also tell us how large or small the real effect might be and yet still give us the observed findings by chance. This additional information is very helpful in allowing us to interpret both borderline significance and non-significance.

Confidence intervals from large studies tend to be quite narrow in width showing the confidence with which the study is able to estimate the size of any real effect. In contrast, confidence intervals from smaller studies are usually wide — showing that the findings are compatible with a wide range of effect sizes.

Although confidence intervals are helpful in providing further information to aid interpretation this interpretation still requires care. The same caveats that apply to p-values (ie. the problems of Type I and Type II errors) apply with equal force to confidence intervals.

Generalisability and particularisation

For all the complexity of understanding bias and chance in the interpretation of the findings from clinical trials another important consideration should not be forgotten. The findings from any given study relate to the patients included in that study. Even if an effect is assessed as (probably) real and large enough to be clinically important, a further question remains. How well are the findings generalisable to other groups of patients and do they particularise to a given individual? P-values and confidence intervals are of no help with this judgement. Assessment of this external validity is made based on the patients' characteristics and the setting and conduct of the trial.

Conclusion

P-values and confidence intervals are both aids to interpretation. Neither gives a complete answer and even using their guidance erroneous judgements can still be made (real effects may go unseen, or effects may be seen where in reality none exist). A clear understanding of the information content of p-values and confidence intervals greatly assists the interpretation of research findings.

Confidence intervals are preferable to p-values as they give a clear idea of the range of true effect sizes which are compatible with the study findings. However, no matter how big the sample, small the p-values or narrow the confidence intervals, the presence of serious bias will always undermine confidence in the findings. P-values and confidence intervals are predicated on the assumption of unbiased study design and execution.

Key points

* Bias must be assessed before p-values and confidence intervals can be interpreted. Even very large samples and very small p-values can mislead if they come from biased studies.

* P-values tell us how likely the results are to have arisen by chance if there is really no effect (and assuming that there is no bias).

* Non-significance does not mean no effect. Small studies will frequently report non-significance even when there are real, important effects.

* Statistical significance does not necessarily mean that the effect is real: by chance alone about one in twenty significant findings will be spurious.

* Statistical significance does not necessarily mean clinically important. It is the size of the effect that determines the importance, not the size of the p-value.

* Confidence intervals are preferable to p-values as they tell us the range of possible effect sizes compatible with the data.

References

Altman DG, Bland JM (1995) Absence of evidence is not evidence of absence. *Br Med J* **311**: 485

Brennan P, Croft P (1994) Interpreting the results of observational research: chance is not such a fine thing. *Br Med J* **309**: 727–30

Crombie IK (1996) *The Pocket Guide to Critical Appraisal*. BMJ Publishing, London

Eypasch E, Lefering R, Kum CK, Troidl H (1995) Probability of adverse events that have not yet occurred: a statistical reminder. *Br Med J* **311**: 619–20

Florey CV (1993) Sample size for beginners. *Br Med J* **306**: 1181–4

Gardner MJ, Altman DG (1986) Confidence intervals rather than p-values: estimation rather than hypothesis testing. *Br Med J* **292**: 746–50

7

Separating association from causation

Huw Davies, Fiona Williams

Health care professionals need to be able to distinguish causal relationships from simple associations in two main areas: when unravelling the aetiology of diseases, and when assessing the effects of therapies. In each of these the presence of confounding can seriously mislead. This chapter explains the nature of confounding and outlines criteria that can be applied to help distinguish causality from mere statistical associations.

The notion of 'cause' lies at the heart of health care. Without an understanding of cause and effect, diseases are unexplained, interventions and outcomes remain unconnected, and effective action is impossible. Making sense of causal relationships is a prerequisite for being an effective practitioner. In addition, researchers and health professionals might be interested in more general examples of effectiveness; such as whether particular organisational configurations function well, or whether certain post-qualification educational experiences are worthwhile. Understanding causal linkages is an essential skill here also.

Health care professionals are largely preoccupied with two specific sorts of causal relationships: those that inform the progression of health problems (disease aetiology); and those that inform their remedy (therapeutic efficacy). This chapter will be concerned with exploring these specific causal relationships, but the comments made are germane to the interpretation of all types of causal linkages.

What is causation?

At its simplest, a cause is something that brings about an effect. But this simplicity hides a variety of different forms of causal relationship. Four basic types can be identified: necessary causes, sufficient causes, necessary and sufficient causes, and neither necessary nor sufficient causes (Elwood, 1992). Necessary causes are those which must be present for a given effect to be observed. For example, infection with herpes zoster is a necessary cause of the chronic condition post-herpetic neuralgia. However, it is not a sufficient cause, as not everyone with herpes zoster infection will go on to develop post-herpetic neuralgia. Sufficient causes are conceptually simple: a given outcome is certain to follow a sufficient cause. However, in health care, non-trivial examples of 'sufficient causes' are unusual: even the most dangerous pathogens spare a few lucky individuals; even the most effective remedies are not infallible.

If sufficient causes are rare, then it is even more unusual in health care for causes to be both sufficient and necessary, that is, where the cause always leads to the effect and the effect never occurs without the presence of the cause. Yet, erroneously, this is how people sometimes conceive of causal relationships — as fixed, deterministic and invariant. Far more usual is for causes to be neither sufficient nor necessary. That is, the cause may be present but the effects may be absent, or the outcomes (we can hardly call them 'effects' in this case) may be seen in the absence of the cause. How then is this a 'causal relationship' at all? The answer lies in whether or not the application of the cause increases the likelihood of the effect. That is, whether there is a statistical relationship (usually called an 'association') between the presence of the cause and the presence of the outcome.

Herein lies the source of much confusion: the presence of a statistical relationship is neither necessary nor sufficient to impute a causal relationship. An association between two variables does not establish that these variables are causally related. Also (but, more rarely) two variables may truly be causally related but a (statistical) association may not readily be apparent.

Association is not causation

'Association is not causation' could be tattooed over the heart of many an epidemiologist. Health professionals could also benefit, not just from knowing this mantra, but also from truly understanding its implications. Most of the causal relationships in health (the causes of diseases and the effectiveness of treatments) are far from deterministic. Identifying links between cause and effect usually consists of first identifying an association and then trying to figure out whether this association reflects a deeper causality.[2] But what is the difference between association and causation?

An association between cause and effect (or outcome) exists if the effect (or outcome) is more common when the putative cause is present than when it is not; an association being a statistical relationship between two variables. If manipulation of the application of the putative cause changes the subsequent frequency of outcome, then that association is deemed causal. An example illustrates the point.

People who carry matches are at increased risk of developing lung cancer. This is a statistical association. However it would be perverse to say that carrying matches causes lung cancer, as any changes to match-carrying habits alone would leave the likelihood of contracting cancer unchanged. People who smoke are also at increased risk of developing lung cancer — yet going beyond this association to call the relationship 'causal' seems warranted, not least because of the evidence that people who change their smoking habits also change their subsequent health risks (Royal College of Physicians, 1971).

Confounded confounding

Assessing the relationship between two variables is complicated. The variables can appear related not because of any causal link but because each is separately related to a third factor. This is called confounding. Consider the example above — people who carry matches are at increased risk of developing lung cancer. Yet carrying matches and lung cancer only appear to be closely related (a statistical association) because each is closely linked to a third factor: smoking itself. In this case smoking is called a confounding variable.

A second example is the paradoxical finding that people who can swim are more likely to drown than those who cannot. Such an association between swimming ability and subsequent drowning seems to throw in doubt the value of swimming lessons. However, a moment's reflection suggests that perhaps those who cannot swim

2   Sometimes, a causal relationship may exist but the association between cause and effect may not readily be apparent. This can happen for the same reason that an association may not reflect causality: namely confounding. For example, a new effective treatment given only to sicker patients may appear no better than standard therapy simply because it is used only on sicker individuals.

steer clear of water in general and water sports in particular. The apparent relationship (a real statistical association) may be less important than at first sight — a possible explanation is variation in a third variable 'propensity to go near deep water' (the confounder). Many apparent relationships (associations) may diminish in interest and importance when the full range of confounding factors is considered.

The examples given were chosen precisely because any causal relationships are implausible and the confounders are obvious. They provide easy illustrations of confounding. In practice, confounders are rarely so conspicuous. Sometimes the postulated relationship may be superficially plausible or even attractive — and an uncritical or inexperienced reader may fail to consider alternative explanations. A further difficulty is that descriptions of empirical associations are rarely provided in a neutral manner. For example, reports of associations between diet and health may assert that 'consumption of produce X reduces disease Y by 20%'; reports of treatment success might similarly claim that 'patients having the new treatment have fewer side-effects and better outcomes'. Such phrasing (for example, using the present tense) may encourage assumptions of causality when the data themselves confirm only past associations. Whether causality can be inferred is an altogether trickier question.

Criteria for causality

Deciding what is causal and what is not has a long history in epidemiology. Over 100 years ago Koch described a set of 'postulates' for determining whether an infectious agent was the cause of a malady (Koch, 1880; Koch 1886). These helped greatly in unravelling the aetiology of infectious disease. Of wider applicability are the criteria identified in the 1960s by the celebrated epidemiologist Sir Austin Bradford Hill (Hill, 1965). These outline a number of considerations for those attempting to identify relationships as causal. Although the criteria have been expanded and at times criticised (Elwood, 1992; Weed, 1997) they nonetheless form a useful framework for thinking about the possible interpretation of empirical associations.

Temporal relationship

That causes should precede effects is axiomatic. When the evidence for any association comes from prospective studies (prospective cohorts or trials for example), such a temporal relationship may be obvious. However, when the data come from retrospective cohorts, case-control studies, cross-sectional studies or case-reports then this relationship may not be so apparent. A lack of the correct time sequence (causes preceding effects) may be enough to reject outright any notion of causality.

Strength

The strength of any association between putative cause and effect (or outcome) is sometimes seen as an indication of the likelihood of causality. Large effect sizes (say three or more for odds ratios or relative risks; see *Chapter 5* and Davies *et al*, 1998) do not of themselves guarantee causality but they do mean that any confounding relationship or bias has to be at least as big. Hopefully, such large biases would be relatively easy to uncover.

Dose-response relationship

A more sophisticated judgement of the strength of any association is whether or not the relationship becomes stronger as more of the putative cause is applied. A classic example is the relationship between carboxyhaemoglobin in the blood and subsequent health outcomes (Beaglehole, 1993). Low levels of carboxyhaemoglobin (say 20%) are associated with mild headache. However, the outcomes become progressively more severe as the percentage increases. At levels of 50% nausea and blackouts are experienced; at 70% unconsciousness ensues; over 80% and death is the most likely result.

Although the presence of a dose-response relationship is often taken as supportive of a causal relationship there are definite reasons to be cautious. For example, the presence of a powerful confounder that has a strong dose-response relationship with the putative cause may produce an apparent dose-response relationship between that cause and the outcome of interest. Crucially, the absence of a dose-response relationship does not prove the absence of any causal relationship. For example, the cause may only operate above a certain threshold, having a step-wise relationship with the outcome, rather than a gradually increasing effect. Alternatively, the association may be U-shaped or J-shaped, such as that between alcohol consumption and cardiovascular disease (Kemm, 1993; Shaper *et al*, 1988). Here, there is a dose-response relationship but only within certain ranges of the cause (alcohol consumption).

Plausibility

That a causal relationship should be plausible is intuitively sensible, but plausibility is limited by the contemporaneous knowledge base. For instance, in the nineteenth century, when Oliver Wendell Holmes first proposed that contagion was responsible for puerperal sepsis many sceptics dismissed this as simply implausible (Holmes, 1842–3). That Holmes was right should serve as a stark warning of the limitations of this requirement. Nonetheless, when coming to some judgement as to whether an observed statistical association reflects an underlying causality, there is no doubt that plausibility is highly influential.

Judgements of plausibility reflect an assessment about how reasonable the findings of an association are in the light of what else is known, especially about biological mechanisms. Postulating a causal relationship between smoking and lung cancer gains credence because of known carcinogens in tobacco smoke that are in contact with lung tissue.

Equally important is the fact that plausibility may provide erroneous support for specious relationships. This is particularly true when it comes to assessing treatments. There are many examples of therapies once thought efficacious but now recognised as of doubtful value (Crombie and Davies, 1996): the surface plausibility of treatments such as radical mastectomy for breast cancer, and neuroablation for chronic pain, wrongly convinced many of their efficacy. Of course, as critics of Oliver Wendell Holmes discovered, a lack of plausibility may also be shaky grounds for rejecting causality.

Consistency

Any substantial causal relationship (factors causing disease, or treatments providing relief) might be expected to have consistency across different individuals and places. When associations are seen only in specific subgroups (defined by age, gender, ethnicity, disease severity or whatever), and there is no substantive biological rationale for the different effects in the sub-groups, then we would quite reasonably suspect that the relationship was artefactual. Again, this criterion provides no hard-and-fast guidance, but a consistent relationship between a cause and an effect seen in different studies conducted on different study populations at different times is reasonably seen as supportive of the belief that the relationship is indeed causal.

Reversibility

A crucial aspect of any relationship between a putative cause and a supposed effect is that manipulation of the cause is followed by changes in the frequency of the effect. Therefore, evidence that removing a cause is associated with a diminution of the effect can be taken as supportive that the relationship is indeed causal. This criterion is again not without problems, once more because of confounding. It is feasible that, unless there is true control over which individuals avoid the putative cause, those choosing to avoid it would in any case be less susceptible to the outcome.

Specificity

A final criterion is that of specificity: that is, the cause should produce specific rather than generalised effects. This is relevant to infectious diseases where, for example, the cholera vibrio produces only cholera. However, the concept is not particularly helpful when considering non-infectious diseases where disease causation is mostly multi-factorial and when causes often produce an array of different health outcomes. Smoking, for example, can cause cancers of the lung, larynx and nose, as well as contributing to cardiovascular disease (Wynder, 1988).

Guidance not guarantees

Given the number of caveats associated with each of the criteria it is clear that although these issues are frequently headlined 'causal criteria' they serve much more usefully as a framework for thinking about the extent of the evidence. None of the above provide incontrovertible support for causality although the first (the temporal relationship) may allow its rejection. Their importance lies in their usefulness as a structure for both research enquiry and study interpretation.

Chance variability

The findings from all studies are subject to the play of chance. That is, any observed association may be a spurious finding due simply to random variability. A substantial real relationship may appear weak or even non-existent for the same reason. Assessment of either of these two possibilities can only occur once spurious systematic reasons for the relationship (biases) have been discounted (Brennan and Croft, 1994). At the very least, reported measures of association (usually relative risk, odds ratio or number-needed-to-treat; see *Chapter 5*) should be surrounded by a confidence interval to aid interpretation (*Chapter 6*).

Sources of evidence

Evidence for causal relationships comes from a range of different study designs — each with its own strengths and weaknesses. The first crucial difference between designs is whether the investigator had experimental control over which individuals were exposed to the putative cause. Exposing people to harmful causes is unethical so this type of study is limited to assessing the benefits of interventions. Randomised controlled trials provide the strongest evidence in support of causal relationships, primarily because the randomisation controls for both known and unknown confounding variables (Cassens, 1992).

When the investigator is unable to control who gets exposed to the putative cause and who does not, the study is said to be observational in design. Observational studies provide weaker evidence than experimental studies but are, nonetheless, the only ethical approach when assessing the causative agents of disease. In all observational studies the presence of confounding is the biggest bugbear. Even within the observational framework different study designs are available and again they have different strengths and weaknesses. Prospective cohort studies tend to provide more robust evidence than either retrospective cohort studies or case-control designs (Abramson, 1984). Simple cross-sectional studies (surveys) are particularly weak at assessing causality, as they may be unable to clarify the temporal relationship between different variables.

Any assessment of causality needs to take account of the inherent weaknesses of the design of the empirical studies that suggest such a relationship. In addition, the actual execution of any study may be flawed, introducing further possibilities of bias. Critical appraisal of study quality should be added to the criteria outlined above. Established tools for carrying out such an appraisal, specific to the different study designs, can ease this task (see *Chapters 11, 13, 14* and *15*, as well as Crombie, 1996; Sackett *et al*, 1991; Sackett *et al*, 1997).

Conclusions

Statistical associations abound but may not reflect meaningful causal relationships. The presence of confounding should always be suspected and creative reflection on any reported association may suggest many plausible confounding variables. Bradford Hill's criteria for assessing causality offer a useful framework for thinking about the presence of causality but they provide no firm guarantees. Also useful are a number of critical appraisal checklists for assessing the various study types that may lead to claims of causal linkages.

Key points

* Association is not causation: a statistical association should not be thought of as a causal relationship without considering whether or not manipulation of the putative cause will lead to changes in the frequency of the specified effect.

* Confounding occurs when any two variables appear to be related because each is separately related to a third (the confounding variable).

* Confounding can hide a true causal relationship or can suggest one when none is present.

* Consideration of a number of criteria can help establish the presence of causality. Foremost among these are that: the putative cause should precede the effect; the relationship between the putative cause and supposed effect should exhibit a 'dose-response' relationship (more of the cause leading to more of the effect); the relationship should be consistent across study groups.

* Causality criteria such as those of Bradford Hill offer a framework for thinking about causality. They do not provide guarantees about its presence or absence.

* Assessment of any biases such as confounding needs to take place before the assessment of the play of chance.

* Different study designs have different strengths in assessing causality. Experimental control can remove problems of confounding which are always present in observational studies. Even so, all studies may be flawed in design, execution and analysis and should be subject to rigorous critical appraisal.

References

Abramson JH (1984) *Survey Methods in Community Medicine: an introduction to epidemiological and evaluative studies.* Churchill Livingstone, Edinburgh

Beaglehole R, Bonita R, Kjellstrom T (1993) *Basic Epidemiology.* World Health Organization, Geneva: 126

Brennan P, Croft P (1994) Interpreting the results of observational research: chance is not such a fine thing. *Br Med J* **309**: 727–30

Cassens BJ (1992) *Preventive Medicine and Public Health.* 2nd edn. National Medical Series. Williams and Wilkins, Baltimore

Crombie IK (1996) *The Pocket Guide to Critical Appraisal.* BMJ Publishing, London

Crombie IK, Davies HTO (1996) *Research in Health Care: design conduct and interpretation of health services research.* John Wiley & Sons, Chichester

Davies HTO, Crombie IK, Tavakoli M (1998) When can odds ratios mislead? *Br Med J* **316**: 689–91

Elwood JM (1992) *Causal Relationships in medicine. A practical system for critical appraisal.* Oxford Medical Publications, Oxford

Hill AB (1965) *The Environment and Disease: association or causation?* Proceedings of the Royal Society of Medicine: Section of Occupational Medicine

Holmes OW (1842–3) The contagiousness of puerperal fever. *N Eng J Med Surg* **1**: 503–30

Kemm J (1993) Alcohol and heart disease: the implications of the U-shaped curve. *Br Med J* **307**: 1373–4

Koch R (1880) *The Aetiology of Traumatic Infective Diseases.*Translated by W Watson Cheyne. New Sydenham Society, London: 21

Koch R (1886) The aetiology of tuberculosis, translated by S Boyd. In: Watson C (ed) *Microparasites in Disease.* New Sydenham Society, London: 65

Royal College of Physicians (1971) *Smoking and Health Now.* Pitman Medical and Scientific Publishing Company Limited, London

Sackett DL, Haynes RB, Guyatt GH, Tugwell P (1991) *Clinical Epidemiology: A Basic Science for Clinical Medicine.* Little, Brown and Company, Boston, Massachusetts

Sackett DL, Richardson WS, Rosenberg W, Haynes RB (1997) *Evidence-based Medicine: how to practice and teach EBM.* Churchill Livingstone, London

Shaper AG, Wannamethee G, Walker M (1988) Alcohol and mortality in British men: explaining the U-shaped curve. *The Lancet* **ii**: 1267–73

Weed DL (1997) On the use of causal criteria. *Int J Epidemiol* **26**: 1137–41

Wynder EL (1988) Tobacco and health: a review of the history and suggestions for public health policy. *Public Health Rep* **103**: 8–18

8

Interpreting reported health care benefits

Aileen Neilson, Huw Davies

When reading published reports on the benefits of different treatments or health care programmes, readers are generally interested in judging the applicability of the results to their own settings. Thus they need to be able to identify what consequences (and costs) were included in the evaluation. This chapter describes the different categories of 'benefit' that may arise from health care interventions and explains some of the methodological considerations in their measurement. It provides simple advice on avoiding the common pitfalls when interpreting the value offered by a particular treatment or configuration of health services.

Empirical data are increasingly being sought on the benefits of treatments and health services. Intuitively the objectives and the resultant 'benefits' of health care may appear rather obvious — to reduce mortality and morbidity from disease (or sometimes simply to reduce costs while maintaining health gains). However, when reviewing evidence from published research reports, the benefits reported may be restricted to a certain type or a particular viewpoint. Such restrictions have the potential to mislead.

In this chapter we describe the nature of 'benefit' in health care studies and indicate the main types of benefits which tend to be included in economic evaluations. In addition, we outline the main methods of analysis and approaches to valuation, the aim being to identify common pitfalls when interpreting benefit data. This paper complements the next chapter explaining health care costs. Detailed checklists for assessing economic studies have already been reported elsewhere (Drummond *et al,* 1996; Jefferson *et al,* 1996).

What is benefit?

We are interested in those services and treatments which deliver more good than harm. Hence an understanding of some basic elements of 'benefit' with respect to health services is necessary if reported studies are to be interpreted correctly.

The consequences of different health care interventions or programmes can be identified with respect to their resulting health effects, the utility (or value) of those effects, and their cost consequences. Which of these are included indicates the perspective of the analysis, ie. who is benefiting from the treatment or programme? The focus could be simply the patient, the patient and the carer, the health service or even society at large.

Effects

The effects of health care interventions are typically described in terms of changes in morbidity and mortality. Studies which are confined to the consideration of health effects are interested in the impact of treatment in terms of changes in the ability of patients to function physically, socially or emotionally. Sometimes this interest is extended to examining changes in patients' families or carers. Studies focusing on health effects assess efficacy or effectiveness and produce standard measures of effect size such as the number needed to treat (NNT) or relative risk reduction (*Chapter 5*).

Utility: quality of life

Not only are the quality of life effects of different treatments and interventions important but the significance or value that patients and their families attach to these effects is also crucial. This valuation of health effects is usually termed their 'utility'. Putting valuations on health changes is highly subjective, practically difficult and sometimes controversial.

Cost consequences

The effects of health care may also be described as changes in resource utilisation. For example, an effective screening programme may uncover latent disease never destined to impact on the health service (thereby raising treatment costs), or it may avert potential future costs associated with the treatment of advanced disease. If the perspective of the analysis is the NHS, then these cost consequences may mean a future benefit (savings) or burden (future cost incurred).

A further (indirect) cost consequence is the impact that treatment may have on patients' ability to perform useful work. A treatment which enables patients to return to work offers benefits to society which should be taken into account. Papers which take a narrow view of benefit may omit some of these potential gains.

The benefits which arise from a treatment or programme may be positive or negative, and are much broader than simply shifts in patients' status (mortality and morbidity). Benefits may encompass the valuations individuals place on health outcomes as well as the cost consequences (both good and bad) of improved treatment.

Estimating benefits

The selection of appropriate units of health care benefit will depend on which of the three categories of benefit are of interest in a specific evaluation.

Measuring effects

Effects are typically measured in natural units and refer only to an individual's ability to function and not to the significance, preference or value attached to this ability. Common measures of effectiveness relating to mortality and morbidity include life-years gained, deaths prevented, pain or symptom free days, cases successfully diagnosed, complications avoided, cases treated appropriately. Some effects relating to morbidity may be measured using generic health status instruments (measuring physical, social or emotional functioning) and/or disease specific instruments. In recent years many health status or health-related quality of life scales have been developed. For example the Nottingham Health Profile (NHP) and the Short Form 36 (SF-36, so called because of its 36 questions) have been used widely in the UK (Bowling, 1995).

Measuring utility

The consequences of alternative treatments or services may also be measured and compared with respect to the (subjective) value of specific levels of health status (utilities). These utilities are derived from the preferences of individuals or society for any particular set of health outcomes. Such preferences are usually expressed on a scale from zero (equivalent to death) to one (equivalent to perfect health). Techniques for measuring utility include simple rating scales, or more complex approaches, such as the 'standard gamble' or 'time trade-off' methods (Torrance, 1986). Each approach generates an adjustment factor with which to increase or decrease the value of time spent in health states. The most common result of utility analyses are quality adjusted life-years (QALYs). Readers should be aware that many issues surrounding QALYs remain unresolved (Neumann *et al*, 1997). For example, it is well documented that there can exist considerable discrepancies between the patient's valuations and those assigned by health-care providers or the general public. (Sprangers and Aaronson, 1992).

Measuring cost consequences

The cost consequences of health care interventions are typically recorded in terms of changes in resource utilisation, for example, numbers of procedures performed, equipment costs, amounts of time or space used and so on. Changes in patients' costs might also be included, measured in terms of the quantity of medication purchased or the number of clinic visits (valued in money terms). Valuation of return-to-work or other indirect benefits (such as time saved) may use average wage rates. There are many pitfalls in estimating costs which are described in *Chapter 9*.

Using measures of benefit — making comparisons

The health benefits (outputs) from treatments or programmes mean very little on their own without some consideration of the inputs used in their generation. Undertaking economic evaluation studies in which the costs and consequences of alternative treatments and health services are compared simultaneously allows us to address questions of efficiency (ie. are the interventions worth the costs?).

The benefits of primary interest indicate the type of economic evaluation being performed. Where costs are compared with measures of effect, a cost-effectiveness analysis is being performed; when valuations in the form of utilities are assigned to those effects then this is called a cost-utility analysis. Finally, if the utilities are converted to monetary values — and all the cost-consequences are included — then this is a cost-benefit analysis.

Cost-effectiveness analysis

When the consequences of two health care interventions (or services) are identical in all relevant respects, our efficiency comparison will be made simply on the basis of cost. However, this type of evaluation — cost-minimisation analysis — requires evidence that outcome differences of the alternatives are either non-existent or unimportant. More usually, there will be differences in the benefits arising from the alternative interventions. In this case, cost-effectiveness analysis compares the benefits of alternative procedures with respect to some common measures of effectiveness. Efficiency questions are then addressed by assessing the results in terms of cost per unit of effect, eg. the cost per life year gained, cost per case cured, or cost per diagnosis.

Cost-utility analysis

In cost-utility analysis, programme effects are translated into a measure of value (utility) based on preferences for health states. A given set of treatment outcomes are adjusted for the utility attached to those outcomes, providing a common denominator for comparison of outcomes and costs in different programmes. To calculate the number of QALYs (the most commonly used utility unit) resulting from a particular intervention, the number of additional years of life gained are combined with a measure of the quality of life in each of these years to obtain a composite index of outcome. For example, two years of life with a utility of 0.5 equates to a single QALY. Comparisons are then based on differences between alternative treatment strategies in the marginal cost per QALY gained.

Cost per QALY 'league tables' have been produced for a host of different treatments and health care services with the aim of guiding decisions on resource allocation (eg. hip replacement, breast cancer screening, or heart and kidney transplantation) (Mason *et al*, 1993). However, a recent review of 86 studies using QALYs found that there was considerable variation in the construction of the QALYs, and that most studies did not adhere to recommended analytical principles (Neumann *et al*, 1997). Studies which generate 'cost-per-QALY' data may not be directly comparable, having been conducted at different times, using different approaches to measure health status or covering different categories of cost. Other arguments against the use of QALYs include allegations that they discriminate against older people, make inappropriate interpersonal comparisons, ignore equity considerations and introduce bias into quality of life scores (Gerard and Mooney, 1993).

Cost-benefit analysis

Cost-benefit analysis extends cost-utility analysis by expressing both the inputs and outputs of treatments and programmes in monetary terms. This requires translating treatment benefits such as QALYs, the prevention of medical complications or the avoidance of disability days, into their monetary benefit. It then becomes possible to say whether a particular procedure or programme offers an overall net gain to society in the sense that its total benefits exceed its total costs.

The two main methods of benefit estimation and valuation are the 'human capital approach' and techniques based on individuals' observed or stated preferences (typically 'willingness to pay' surveys) (Sugen and Williams, 1979; Drummond, 1981). The human capital approach measures the benefits of health care (eg. avoidable morbidity and mortality) in terms of the future flow of income that would otherwise be foregone because of ill health. The 'willingness to pay' approach seeks to establish the value that people attach to health outcomes by asking them how much they (hypothetically) would be prepared to pay to obtain the benefits of care or avoid the costs of illness.

Both approaches are open to criticism. The 'human capital' approach sees people's worth solely in terms of their earning power. This diminishes the worth of the unemployed, the retired, home-makers and children. It also downplays the importance of the non-financial aspects of ill-health such as pain, suffering, loss and grief. However, estimating the value of benefits using 'willingness to pay' surveys is also problematic. The valuations obtained can be sensitive to the way in which questions are asked and tend to be related to respondents' income. Thus, converting 'benefits' to a monetary value is certainly no exact science. A clear understanding of how values were obtained is needed before findings can be judged reasonable.

Although studies generally state which economic evaluation approach is being used it is important to check whether this is indeed the case. A recent review of 95 studies labelled as cost-benefit evaluations and appraised against standard definitions of this technique revealed that 53% were actually only partial evaluations because health gains were not properly evaluated (Zarnke *et al*, 1997).

Benefit now or benefit later?

It is part of human nature to want our benefits now and our costs deferred. Because of this, some would argue that both costs and benefits obtained some way into the future are worth less than they would be if obtained in the present. This reduction in value into the future is called 'discounting'.

The traditional view has been that future benefits should be discounted in the same way as future costs, although arguments have been advanced both for and against such a move (Cairns, 1992; Parsonage and Neuberger, 1992). What is of importance to the reader is not whether we should or should not discount benefits, but what are the consequences for the main study findings if one view is adopted over another. Discounting benefits means that procedures with long lasting effects such as neonatal care, maternity services, health prevention and promotion activities — which lead to benefits over the recipient's entire future lifetime — receive lower priority. Not discounting benefits would change the relative cost-effectiveness of different procedures and make projects with long lasting effects relatively more cost-effective.

Sensitivity analysis

Users of economic evaluations will be interested to know how robust the initial results are to variations in the values of the key estimates and assumptions used. For example, the size of any treatment effect may vary between patient groups as may the costs incurred. Reporting such 'sensitivity analyses' enables readers to consider to what extent the authors have allowed for uncertainties inherent in their analysis. This is not always done in published work: a recent methodological review of published cost-effectiveness and cost-benefit analyses found that many evaluations failed to make underlying assumptions explicit and failed to test assumptions with sensitivity analyses (Briggs and Sculpher, 1995).

Conclusion

Studies which report on the benefits of treatments and services require the reader to be familiar with some of the important elements of appropriate evaluation techniques. Many difficulties arise in measuring, let alone valuing, the benefits arising from health care interventions. It is impossible to judge the headline findings from economic analyses without a detailed assessment of all the individual judgements or estimates made along the way. In addition, it is important to check the data sources used for the analysis — data may be suspect for either inputs or outputs, and the conclusions of any analysis are only as good as the underlying studies used to estimate the base data. Even so, because of the uncertainty associated with these issues, thorough sensitivity analyses exploring the robustness of the conclusions are an essential factor in building confidence in the findings.

Key points

* The outputs of health care may be reported in terms of their health effects, the utility (or value) of those effects, or their cost consequences.

* Cost-effectiveness analysis (CEA), cost-utility analysis (CUA) and cost-benefit analysis (CBA) are methods of economic evaluation used to measure and compare the economic costs and consequences associated with alternative programmes and procedures.

* CEA measures consequences in terms of natural units, such as cost per life year saved, cost per case cured, or cost per symptom-free day.

* CUA expresses outcomes as a single utility-based unit of measurement, for example, the quality adjusted life year (QALY).

* In CBA, monetary values are placed on both the inputs (costs) and the outcomes (benefits) of health care to give an overall estimation of net monetary benefit.

* Ideally, cost-effectiveness studies should be built-in alongside clinical trials, or should draw on published data. In the absence of data, any assumptions must be made explicit.

* Sensitivity analyses should be applied when there is uncertainty about the effectiveness (and costs) of different procedures to investigate the extent to which results are sensitive to alternative assumptions about key variables.

* The discounting of benefits is controversial although most economic evaluations do choose to do this.

References

Bowling A (1995) *Measuring Disease: A review of disease specific quality of life measurement scales.* Open University Press, Buckingham

Briggs A, Sculpher M (1995) Sensitivity analysis in economic evaluation: a review of published studies. *Health Econ* 4(5): 355–371

Cairns J (1992) Discounting and health benefits. Another perspective. *Health Econ* 1: 76–79

Drummond MF (1981) Welfare economics and cost-benefit analysis in healthcare. *Scott J Political Econ* 28(2): 125–145

Drummond MF, Stoddart GL, Torrance GW (1996) *Methods for the economic evaluation of healthcare programmes.* Oxford University Press, Oxford

Gerard K, Mooney G (1993) QALY league table: handle with care. *Health Econ* 2(1): 59–64

Jefferson T, Demicheli V, Mugford, M (1996) *Elementary economic evaluation in health care.* BMJ Publishing Group, London

Mason J, Drummond M, Torrance G (1993) Some guidelines on the use of cost-effectiveness league tables. *Br Med J* 306: 570–572

Neumann PJ, Zinner DE, Wright JC (1997) Are methods for estimating QALYs cost-effectiveness analyses improving? *Med Decis Making* 17(4): 402–408

Parsonage M, Neuberger H (1992) Discounting and health benefits. *Health Econ* 1: 71–76

Sprangers MAG, Aaronson NK (1992) The role of health care providers and significant others in evaluating the quality of life of patients with chronic disease: A review. *J Clin Epidemiol* 7: 743–760

Sugden R, Williams AH (1979) *The Principles of Practical Cost-benefit Analysis.* Oxford University Press, Oxford

Torrance GW (1986) Measurement of health state utilities for economic appraisal. *J Health Econ* 5: 1–30

Zarnke KB, Levine MA, O'Brien BJ (1997) Cost-benefit analyses in the health-care literature: don't judge a study by its label. *J Clin Epidemiol* 50(7): 813–822

9

Interpreting reported health care costs

Aileen Neilson, Huw Davies

In addition to assessing evidence of treatment effectiveness, evaluating cost implications is growing in importance. Many published research reports now attempt to assess the costs of different treatment options. But how can information on treatment costs be interpreted? Published reports are not always clear in their definition of 'costs', and may be reticent about the 'rules' used in cost measurement. Making comparisons between studies is only possible when we are confident that we understand the cost estimation process and are sure that we are comparing like with like. This chapter describes the different categories of costs and methodological considerations in cost measurement. It provides simple advice on avoiding some of the common pitfalls in cost interpretation and should help readers in assessing the usefulness of reported costs.

A considerable amount of evidence is being generated on the economic impact of different diagnostic and therapeutic interventions. Doctors not only face the task of reading and appraising evidence of clinical effectiveness but they must also be able to understand and interpret evidence of the comparative costs of alternative treatments and health service configurations. Studies which arrive at a statement on the estimated costs of a particular treatment or service should prompt the reader to question how these estimates were derived. Many assumptions are made during cost estimation and, unless these are made explicit and are well understood by the reader, erroneous judgements may be made.

In this chapter we describe the nature of cost in health care studies and highlight the main categories of costs. A brief discussion of the key methodological issues emphasises the hidden assumptions which may alter our interpretation of the 'bottom line' figures. Detailed checklists for assessing economic evaluations have already been reported elsewhere (Drummond and Stoddart, 1996; Jefferson *et al*, 1996) and the reader is encouraged to use these in assessing reported studies.

What is cost?

An understanding of some basic economic concepts is necessary if reported costs are to be interpreted correctly. Economics is all about the allocation of scarce resources through the process of comparative analyses and prioritisation of services. In comparing and making choices between different courses of actions we note that costs are incurred in making specific decisions. A decision to have more of something means sacrificing (having less of) something else because we cannot do everything (resources are limited). Thus the 'cost' of pursuing one particular course of action can be thought of not just as the money spent on that option, but more appropriately as the benefits lost because of not choosing the next best alternative. This notion of 'benefits foregone' — because we choose to use resources in one way rather than another — is central to economics. To an economist, cost is less about money spent and more about the value of lost opportunities. When we speak of costs we should think in terms of 'opportunity costs'.

The concept of opportunity cost clarifies that there is an important distinction between the price of health care and its cost. When interpreting studies it is a mistake to regard these two as the same. Prices are frequently notional at best and are often driven by market forces, whereas 'costs' are the (opportunity) cost of production. For example, the published figures in Scottish Health Service Costs (1997) are based mainly on the annual accounts of health boards, NHS trusts and Scottish Financial Returns (mainly hospital running costs and community services). Whether the quoted values are in any way indicative of the value that might be obtained if resources were removed from one service and re-allocated to another is very much in doubt.

Costs to whom?

Each analysis of costs must take a stance on the importance of who is paying specific costs. For example, a cost analysis by a Trust may ignore or downplay costs incurred in primary care, whereas the same analysis by a Health Authority would wish to see these costs accounted for. Studies which are explicit about who pays the costs (and consequently which costs are included) are more helpful than those which leave such an important assumption unstated. Different studies may take different viewpoints from the most inclusive (a societal or health care sector view where almost all costs are covered) through to a more restrictive view (eg. analysis at Trust or even directorate level which may omit costs not immediately borne by the institution or cost centre).

Because different studies may take different viewpoints they may come to markedly different conclusions. For example, calculation of the costs to society of a cancer screening programme will usually include not just the costs of screening and treating, but also the costs to the patient of attendance, and the costs of all morbidity arising from screening and treatment. On the other hand, calculation of costs to a hospital will generally only include those costs borne directly by the hospital, but not costs that patients incur or that society might incur from long-term morbidity. Readers need to identify at the outset the underlying view of the costs analysis and judge the findings accordingly.

Identifying costs

Costs which can be considered for inclusion in a study fall into three main categories: direct costs; indirect costs; and intangible costs.

Direct costs

The first group of costs are known as direct costs and reflect those borne by health services. These costs include both capital and operating costs. Capital costs — purchasing of equipment, buildings and land — represent investments in assets at the beginning of the service which are then used over time. The two components of capital cost are the opportunity cost of the funds tied up in the capital investment and the depreciation over time of the assets themselves. Operating costs cover such things as health professionals' time, supplies and equipment, as well as overhead costs. Overhead costs are resources that serve different departments and programmes, eg. general hospital administration, plant operations and maintenance, materials management, central laundry, medical records, cleaning, porters, power etc. If individual services are to be costed, these shared costs may need to be attributed across different programmes. For example in Scottish Health Service Costs (1997) costs are analysed between direct costs and allocated costs.

It will be immediately apparent that there is much scope for manoeuvre in identifying and allocating these costs. Readers need to check carefully to ensure that all areas have been covered in any given study, or that two studies producing comparative costs have identified direct costs in a similar manner.

Indirect costs

The second category of costs are known as indirect costs. These are costs and productivity losses borne by patients, their families, employers or even society at large. Such costs may include loss in earnings and out-of-pocket expenses (eg. self-medication, travel, opportunity costs of time spent accessing care). Again judgement is used by researchers in identifying which costs to measure and include, and this judgement may affect the bottom line figures.

Intangible costs

Thirdly, the costs of pain, grief and suffering, and the loss of leisure time constitute intangible costs. These costs are often neglected by costing studies because, first, they are hard to identify and measure and, second, they are difficult to value. For example, it may be possible to identify that women given a false positive result from a mammogram will suffer anxiety and distress until given reassurance at follow-up; it may even be possible to quantify that distress to some extent; but it is much more difficult to assign objective value to this 'cost'.

These three categories cover the cost items relevant to most costing analyses of alternative health care programmes or services. It will be readily apparent that it is a complex task to identify, apportion and value all the different components. It should also be clear that different judgements are involved along the way — about what is important and should be included, and what is not and can be ignored. Once the additional judgements involved in valuing intangible costs are included, it is evident that there is great scope for wide variations in the 'bottom line' arising from different (but nonetheless reasonable) approaches to costing.

Estimating the costs

After identifying the important and relevant items to be included in the analysis, costs need to be measured. There are two parts to cost estimation: what are the units of measurement? and how many 'units' have been consumed? Costs need to be measured in appropriate physical units (eg. hours of nursing or consultant time, number of clinic visits, number of days in hospital, number of working days lost). Of particular importance, and a frequent omission in analyses, is how common overheads are measured (eg. laboratory services, utilities, cleaning and administration). There is no single approach to the allocation of resource use to each treatment or service, and studies sometimes use physical units to distribute common costs (eg. number of patients, size of staff, number of square feet). Such approaches may be useful when examining the impact of expansion or contraction of particular programmes on the use of central services.

Market prices are generally used to estimate costs for individual items based on a typical pattern of care (eg. medical staff, commodities and services). However, charges set by the market place may bear little resemblance to the actual cost of providing a product or service (Finkler, 1982). For example, calculation of costs to a hospital (a provider of health care) usually reflect real use of resources from providing the service rather than the charges paid by patients. Therefore some cost finding exercises use quite detailed cost accounting techniques. On the other hand, market prices or charges measure cost only to those who pay those charges (through private health insurance policies and national insurance contributions).

Some of the common pitfalls in this process include the use of inappropriate measures, the failure to dis-aggregate total costs and poor estimation of resource use.

What sort of cost — average, marginal or incremental?

Studies will often report on three different kinds of costs: average, marginal and incremental. The latter two are often confused. The average cost of a particular treatment or programme is obtained by dividing the total cost by the number of units produced. This approach might be used, for example, to estimate the average cost per patient day. This gives a global picture but is uninformative about the costs of change.

The change in total cost resulting from expanding (or reducing) within a particular programme or service is known as the marginal cost. This allows us to understand the implications of an expansion or reduction in services.

Frequently, however, we wish to compare costs between alternative programmes. For this we should use the incremental cost. This is the difference between the marginal costs of the alternative programmes. Of course, it is only meaningful if the costings for the alternative programmes have been calculated in exactly the same way.

Using costs — making comparisons

There are various ways of using cost estimates to make comparisons as a basis for judging value for money or setting priorities. All three categories of cost (average, marginal or incremental) can be combined with measures of effectiveness (eg. cases detected, deaths prevented, life-years gained) to obtain a summary measure of programme efficiency. This is called a cost-effectiveness ratio (Krahn and Gafni, 1993) and it provides an estimate of the cost per unit of benefit of a given programme, service or treatment.

Which of the three categories of cost is used in calculating the cost-effectiveness ratio depends on the purpose of the calculation and makes a great difference to the end result. Problems often arise when the wrong cost estimates are used for making comparisons.

Estimating the cost effectiveness ratio of developing a new service for which there is no alternative provision means that the average costs have to be used. What is being estimated here is a measure of the cost of producing one unit of output that is independent of any other programmes. More usually however, we will be comparing different levels of providing the same service (eg. screening for cancer every three years rather than every five years). In this case, it is inappropriate to use the total costs in the cost effectiveness ratio — marginal costs should be used. These give us some idea of what extra benefit we can gain for what extra cost. To obtain meaningful comparisons between alternative approaches to delivering the same service, we need to examine the incremental costs and then compare these with the additional benefits delivered.

There are various ways in which cost effectiveness ratios can be calculated and which is appropriate depends crucially on the question being tackled. In particular, we should examine reported costings bearing in mind changes, either within a service (expansion or contraction), or movements between alternatives. In this context it is marginal costs and benefits that matter.

Paying now or paying later?

Given the choice of paying now or paying later, most people would choose to pay later. Therefore the timing of costs incurred must be taken into account (Parsonage and Neuberger, 1992). Costing studies should reflect this characteristic of human nature by downplaying costs which will be incurred some time later compared to those which have to be provided up-front. They do this by discounting (or reducing) future costs to reflect their present values. This raises the important question of by how much future costs should be discounted?

Typically, future costs are discounted using a rate of between 2% and 10%. Often the discount rate is based on rates that have been used in other published studies (to facilitate comparisons), or is based on government recommended rates (previously 5%, more recently 6% [Udvarhelyi *et al*,˙ 1992]). If many costs are incurred at some time into the future the choice of discount rate can have a dramatic effect: a large discount rate will tend to underplay these costs. If two programmes are being compared, one with large up-front costs and the other with largely deferred costs, the sensitivity of the findings to different discount rates should be assessed.

Sensitivity analysis

As will be clear by now, estimating costs is a messy business with many assumptions, approximations and guestimates. But does this matter? The key question is whether the bottom line is greatly changed if a different set of assumptions and figures are used. Exploration of how sensitive the final figures are to changes in the constituent parts is called sensitivity analysis. Two key questions to ask of any analysis are:

- was a sensitivity analysis carried out?
- were the findings robust?

A good costings study will be very explicit about the assumptions made, deficiencies in the information sources, valuations proposed and amount of sheer guesswork. It will then attempt to explore whether the final conclusions are sensitive to changes in any of the underlying details. If the bottom line is little changed by even wide fluctuations in its constituent parts then we would call the findings robust and have some confidence that underlying judgements were not critical in affecting the final result. A sensitivity analysis which shows that findings are not robust at least identifies the important factors in determining the bottom line. Readers can then form their own judgement about the important underlying assumptions and draw their own conclusions. Studies without sensitivity analyses leave us unsure about the stability and validity of the findings.

Conclusion

Costing analyses which arrive at a figure for the estimated cost of treatments and services require the reader to be familiar with some of the important elements of good costing exercises. Good quality costing studies should be as explicit as possible about the underlying details which have gone into the final cost estimates. A detailed sensitivity analysis should draw attention to the critical variables and assumptions.

Interpreting costs data, and combining them with measures of effectiveness, requires careful attention to the context of change. The specific question or purpose will determine how costs are compared but changes at the margin will always be of interest.

Key points

* In appraising costing studies, particular attention should be given to what extent the study a) identifies the important and relevant costs, b) accurately estimates the measurement of costs in appropriate physical units, and c) values these costs credibly.

* The variable extent of coverage of direct, indirect and intangible costs is related to the viewpoint of the study and the degree of difficulty in identifying, tracking and estimating costs.

* Costs reported may be derived from charges (often set by the market place) or may use detailed cost accounting techniques; whatever approach is used the reader should try to think in terms of 'opportunity costs'.

* Marginal costs (and benefits) should be used in assessing the impact of contraction or expansion of a service.

* Incremental costs (and benefits) should be used in making comparisons between alternative programmes.

* Future costs should be adjusted to their present day values by discounting.

* Sensitivity analysis demonstrates whether a conclusion is robust over a range of plausible assumptions or whether it hinges on the accuracy of a particular assumption.

* Costing studies do not permit us to answer efficiency questions — cost-effectiveness, cost-utility and cost-benefit analyses are required for this purpose.

References

Drummond MF, Stoddart GL, Torrance GW (1996) *Methods for the Economic Evaluation of Healthcare Programmes*. Oxford University Press, Oxford

Finkler SA (1982) The distinction between cost and charges. *Ann Intern Med* **96**:102–109

Jefferson T, Demicheli V, Mugford M (1996) *Elementary Economic Evaluation in Health Care*. BMJ Publishing Group, London

Krahn M, Gafni A (1993) Discounting in the economic evaluation of health care interventions. *Med Care* **31**(5): 403–418

Parsonage M, Neuberger H (1992) Discounting and health benefits. *Health Econ* **1**: 76–79

Scottish Health Service Costs 1996/97, National Health Service in Scotland, Information and Statistics Division, Edinburgh 1997

Udvarhelyi IS, Colditz GA, Rai A, Epstein AM (1992) Cost-effectiveness and cost-benefit analyses in the medical literature. *Ann Intern Med* **116**: 238–244

Section II:
Issues in research design

10

Bias in surveys

Huw Davies

The simple survey is a regular tool in health services research. But, like any research method, surveys can be flawed in design, execution, analysis or interpretation. This chapter outlines the basis of good survey design and advises how bias in published studies can be assessed.

Surveys are ubiquitous in health care. There are surveys to assess health care need, use or demand; surveys to assess attitudes, beliefs, knowledge and opinions (of health care professionals as well as patients); and surveys to assess the patients' experience of health care encounters. The simple survey is an invaluable tool for gaining insight into patients, health care services or the interactions between the two.

Nonetheless, for all their apparent simplicity, surveys have the power to mislead as well as to inform. Like any research technique, surveys have pitfalls — they can be used inappropriately (for example, to answer questions to which they are ill-suited), or they can be badly designed, poorly executed or erroneously interpreted. This chapter discusses the key design issues upon which surveys stand or fall, and advises on how to assess any flaws in published studies.

Asking the right questions

Surveys have a design that is described as 'cross-sectional'. That is, they take a slice of the world at a given time point. They are ideally suited to quantifying how many individuals have what sort of characteristics and to what extent. Problems arise when some notion of temporality is introduced into the research questions, when we begin to ask about what happened in the past or about how different characteristics are linked. For example, suppose we took a sample of patients with diabetes who are being managed on a new form of insulin. Surveying these patients to discover what they think of the new formulation, and how it compares to their previous experience, may seem like a reasonable thing to do. However, such a survey will fail to capture the experience of individuals who tried the new formulation for only a brief time and then reverted back to their old approach.

A second common pitfall with surveys is the presentation of associations between different characteristics in the hope of shedding light on causal linkages. A previous chapter demonstrated how unsatisfactory it is to make these kinds of assertions from cross-sectional data (*Chapter 7*). Further problems may arise when analyses of subgroups within survey data are used to draw conclusions for which longitudinal data are needed. For example, consider data gathered from a population-based survey on blood cholesterol. Suppose these data show that the average blood cholesterol is lowest in the youngest age group, higher in successive older age groups, and then lower again in those aged over 65. One might be tempted to conclude from this that blood cholesterol increases as we age, but falls off after retirement. This may of course be true, but these data, gathered from a survey, are unable to demonstrate this. It may be, for example, that confounding factors explain the apparent rise (middle-aged people may, for example, have a quite different diet from younger people). Alternatively, it may be the case that people who are in mid-years now had a very different upbringing and have had consistently elevated cholesterol levels all along. Perhaps even the apparent fall-off of cholesterol in the oldest group can be explained by the selective early death of those with abnormally high levels of cholesterol.

What we do not know, and would need to know to draw some conclusions about how cholesterol levels vary with age, is what happens to the surveyed individuals as time unfolds. Following up the individuals in the survey and looking at individual changes in cholesterol level would help to determine which scenario will be played out in practice: will cholesterol fall, rise or remain the same? As soon as we begin to be interested in questions with a temporal component (eg. what happens next and why? or what happened in the past and how does it relate to the present?) then the more appropriate study designs are longitudinal ones, such as cohort studies (*Chapter 11*) and prospective trials (*Chapter 14*).

Representative samples

Assuring that a survey is the appropriate design for the questions being asked is only the first stage in critically appraising a published study. Whatever data are actually gathered and presented in a survey, it is rare that those individuals included in the study are the only individuals of interest. Far more usual is the situation when we want to use the data that we have on some selected individuals to say something interesting and relevant about some other wider group of interest. Sometimes, this wider group of interest has a clearly defined existence (eg. a survey of general practitioners might want to infer something about general practitioners as a whole). At other times, the wider group of interest is more notional — for example, a survey of patients attending for a flu shot might want to draw some conclusions about all such patients, both now and in the immediate future.

That surveys want to make some inferences about wider groups than the individuals actually studied raises some important questions about whether the data collected can support such inferences. In order to be confident that drawing wider conclusions is reasonable, we must first be convinced that the study group are representative of the wider group of interest; that is, they must be similar in all possible ways to the target group. Confirming that this is so can be difficult or even impossible. However, having some knowledge about how the survey was designed and conducted can allow judgements about representativeness to be well-founded. There are two ways in which representativeness can be compromised. First, the survey may be designed in such a way that certain individuals in the wider group of interest have no chance of being included in the study sample. This is called non-coverage. Second, those selected for inclusion in the study can fail to deliver any information. This is called non-response. *Figure 10.1* illustrates where these deficiencies may arise: both may introduce bias. *Chapter 2* also explores these issues in more detail.

Non-coverage

The design of the survey begins with some definition (even informally) of the target group of interest — the notional group about whom data from the survey are designed to provide insight. Next some kind of sampling frame is set up — a list or means of contact from which study subjects will be selected for inclusion. In assessing bias in surveys, the initial questions to ask are:

- which members of the target group might be missing from the sampling frame?
- how might those missing differ from those who are included?

Of course, getting onto the sampling frame is no guarantee that a representative sample will be drawn. To avoid bias requires that a sampling method be chosen which ensures that each member of the sampling frame is equally likely to be selected in the final sample. Simple random sampling is the simplest way of achieving this, but other methods (such as multi-stage sampling) may also be acceptable. Failure at either of these two stages (drawing up the sampling frame, or selecting the sample from the sample frame) may introduce non-coverage bias.

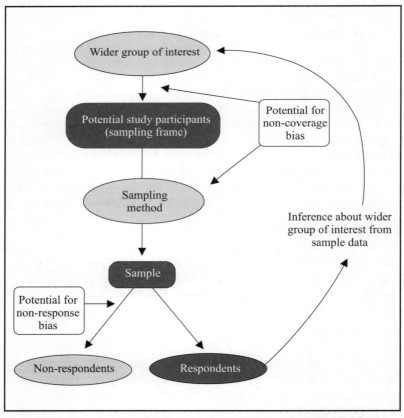

Figure 10.1: From group of interest to survey data: the potential for bias

Non-response

Once a fair sample has been selected the problem still remains of non-response. Individuals contacted may fail to provide data for a range of reasons: they may have died, moved away or even just refuse to participate. As some of these reasons may be connected with the questions being asked in the survey, it is a safe assumption that those who do not reply will differ in many ways from those that do. Non-response may introduce serious bias into the survey findings. For example, those who respond to a survey may well be those who hold strong views on the issue in question — so presenting a false picture.

There is no level at which a response rate becomes respectable — and conversely, no level beneath which the findings are valueless. If the survey is carried out to discover a ballpark figure (many or few? often or rarely?) then even quite low response rates (less than 50%) may still provide useful information. For example, consider a survey with a response rate of 50%, which discovers that 60% of respondents have suffered a hangover. This survey at least places the likely true proportion as being somewhere between 30% and 80% (depending on whether all of the non-respondents have had a hangover or none of them, and subject to additional uncertainty through chance variation — see below). This may be sufficiently precise, or hopelessly imprecise, depending on what was previously known and what use is intended to be made of the survey information.

In contrast, a survey that seeks an accurate estimate of a relatively rare phenomenon may be hopelessly flawed even with a response rate of over 90%. Thus an acceptable level for the response rate depends crucially on the questions being asked.

Measurement problems

Having ascertained that the study sample is not unreasonably biased, the next major consideration is of the quality of the data collected. The questions asked are about the questionnaire or other data-gathering instrument, and any measures used. In essence, we are interested in the data **reliability** and the data **validity**. Reliability is concerned with reassurance that data gathering by different individuals, or at a different time or in a different context, would not yield different findings given no true change in the study participants. Validity, a more elusive concept, is concerned with ensuring that the data presented are in fact measuring what it is intended that they measure. *Chapter 1* provides more detail on these issues.

Simple physical measurements such as height and weight, or factual data gathering such as age, gender and educational attainment, may be relatively unproblematic (although even here there is scope for systematic biases to creep in). However, substantial difficulties arise when attempts are made at measuring complex concepts such as quality of life, psychosocial functioning, or patient satisfaction. Even seemingly relatively straightforward issues such as pain, mobility or symptomatology can hide myriad measurement difficulties. Such measures may be inherently inadequate or flawed, and they are particularly prone to bias arising from the settings in which the data are gathered or the nature of the gathering mechanism. For example, data collected in the home setting may tell a different story from ostensibly the same data collected in a clinical setting. Convincing surveys will go to considerable lengths to reassure that any measurement difficulties have been understood and overcome.

Size matters

All of the above considerations have been about bias in surveys: systematic deviations from the truth introduced during the design, execution, analysis or interpretation. One further problem remains: that of chance variability. As surveys almost invariably present data from samples, any given set of findings is just one of many possible instances. Any findings must be placed in the context of an understanding about how data might vary given the play of chance. This is usually done by creating '95% confidence intervals' around any sample values.

Table 10.1 shows the confidence intervals for a given sample percentage and different sizes of (randomly drawn) samples. There are two things to note from this table. First, samples of under a hundred or so have relatively wide confidence intervals (perhaps ±10% around the sample estimate, and even as much as ±20% for samples of just 25). Second, in order to increase the precision of an estimate from a survey much larger samples are needed. In fact, in order to reduce the confidence interval by half, four times as many individuals are required in the sample. It is only with sample sizes of around 1000 that the confidence interval around a sample estimate is as narrow as ±3%. Again, the level of sample variability acceptable depends on the questions that the survey is being used to answer.

Small samples may be acceptable for rough estimates, but precision requires the use of large samples.

In particular, if a survey finds no instances of a particular feature (a zero percent) this does not necessarily mean that the feature is absent. The zero finding could have been produced by chance alone. A useful statistical approximation is that the confidence interval for a zero finding is from 0% to approximately 300/n % (where n is the survey sample size). This useful approximation holds for samples of about 20 or more (Eypasch *et al*, 1995). A zero percent from a sample of 30 gives an upper confidence interval of about 10%; and a zero from a sample of size 300 still has an upper confidence interval of 1%.

Table 10.1: Confidence intervals (95%) for sample proportions

Proportion in sample	Survey sample size				
	n=25	n=75	n=100	n=200	n=1000
20%	4–36%	11–29%	12–28%	14–26%	17–23%
50%	30–70%	39–61%	40–60%	43–57%	47–53%
80%	64–96%	71–89%	72–88%	74–86%	77–83%

In conclusion

Surveys are easy to design and relatively quick to execute. They are also easy to appraise for flaws. In essence, we are interested in four things:

- are the research questions appropriate for a survey design?
- is the sample group representative?
- are the measures reliable and valid?
- was the sample of sufficient size?

Providing clear answers to these questions should expose any major deficiencies in published studies. More detailed guidance for assessing survey design and analysis can be found in a number of published texts, both for generic surveys (Crombie, 1996) and for surveys with specific design intentions, such as assessing patient satisfaction (Fitzpatrick, 1991). Full explication of the design issues can be found in standard textbooks (Streiner and Norman, 1989; Oppenheim, 1992; Schuman and Presser, 1996).

Key points

* Surveys answer questions about how many? How much? And what sort? They are not readily able to say much about the interrelationships between variables over time.

* The three key questions to ask about a published survey are: Is the sample representative? What was the quality of the measures used in data gathering? And was the sample of sufficient size?

* In assessing representativeness, we should be asking what are the implications for the study findings of both non-coverage and non-response?

* In assessing the quality of the measures used the key issues are reliability (does the measure produce stable answers?) and validity (is the measure providing a true picture of the attributes of interest?).

* Small surveys provide imprecise estimates. Doubling the precision of these estimates requires a four-fold increase in sample size.

References

Crombie IK (1996) *The Pocket Guide to Critical Appraisal.* BMJ Publishing, London

Eypasch E, Lefering R, Kum CK, Troidl H (1995) Probability of adverse events that have not yet occurred: a statistical reminder. *Br Med J* **311**: 619–20

Fitzpatrick R (1991) Surveys of patient satisfaction: I — Important general considerations. *Br Med J* **302**: 887–9

Fitzpatrick R (1991) Surveys of patient satisfaction: II — Designing a questionnaire and conducting a survey. *Br Med J* **302**: 1129–32

Oppenheim AN (1992) *Questionnaire Design, Interviewing and Attitude Measurement.* Pinter Publishers Ltd, London

Schuman H, Presser S (1996) *Questions and Answers in Attitude Surveys.* Sage, Thousand Oaks, CA

Streiner DL, GR Norman (1989) *Health measurement scales: a practical guide to their development and use.* Oxford University Press, Oxford

11

Bias in cohort studies

Huw Davies, Iain Crombie

Cohort studies allow an exploration of patient change over time. They can provide information on the incidence of disease, prognosis (including patient satisfaction) and likely health care resource use. Nonetheless, bias can be present in cohort studies in the way patients are selected and followed up, the way measures are taken, or how data are analysed. This chapter explores ways in which such flaws can be uncovered in published studies, so that their findings can be interpreted appropriately.

Many worthwhile questions in health care involve an exploration of how events unfold over time. What is the incidence of disease? What prognosis can patients expect, and how does this vary depending upon the patients' characteristics and circumstances? What health care services will patients use at different points in their illness? What binds these questions is that they all involve an unfolding picture: attempts to provide answers to these questions therefore involve summarising events over a period of time.

The research design most appropriate to answer these sorts of question is called a cohort study (also known as a follow-up study or a longitudinal design). In essence, a cohort study involves selection of a group of individuals, followed by measurement of some aspects of those individuals on at least two occasions separated by a time interval. Sometimes repeated measures are taken at different intervals widely spaced — in the order of months, years or even decades. In other studies just two measures are taken and the time elapsed might be as short as days or even hours.

The word cohort is derived from the name of a unit of soldiers in a Roman legion: a cohort being a tenth part of a legion. As a cohort of soldiers marches along a road, so study subjects in a cohort study can be thought of as passing through time, from one health state to another. Data collection in a cohort study is then analogous to capturing information on individual soldiers as they pass specific way-markers.

For all the basic simplicity of design, bias can creep into cohort studies in a number of ways. This chapter explores the source of these biases and advises on their identification and assessment.

The right design

Cohort studies are used to explore change, and in answering questions like this they are far superior to surveys (*Chapter 10*). However, analyses reporting changes in individuals are often embedded in survey projects. So the first question to ask of any research reporting relationships over time, is was the design a true cohort with repeated measures on the same sample group collected at different time intervals? If data were in fact collected at only one time point, with patients asked to recollect facts from earlier periods, then the design is a survey not a cohort — and surveys are not well suited to this kind of analysis.

Some research studies report data collected on different groups of individuals collected at distinct time-points, and try to draw conclusions about change. Such a design is again not a cohort study (which involves repeated data collection on the same group of individuals). It is, instead, simply a collection of surveys. Again, the interpretation of data from repeated surveys is problematic.

Even when the study design is a true cohort, it may be poorly suited to answering the research question posed. In particular, assessing whether changes in patient status are causally related to health care activities needs the added design features of a rigorous trial (*Chapter 14*) if the dangers of confounding are to be avoided (*Chapter 7*). For example, cohort studies of the effects of maternal analgesia during childbirth on subsequent behaviour of the baby have found many interesting associations (Lieberman *et al*, 1979). Yet interpretation of these is difficult because of the many maternal factors which influence both choice of maternal analgesia and subsequent baby development. Cohort studies can describe changes and the factors that are associated with these changes; they are less able to explain whether these factors are causal or not (*Chapter 7*).

Sample selection

Cohort studies begin by taking a sample of patients. Many of the issues about representativeness discussed previously on surveys (*Chapters 2 and 10*) are equally germane to the sampling of individuals in cohort studies. Selection bias takes many forms (Sackett, 1979) and can lead to unusual groups and artefactual relationships. For example, samples of patients recruited from specialist clinics will show important differences from those recruited from community settings (Crombie and Davies, 1998). They will tend to have more severe and intractable disease and will have had longer treatment histories. These differences in turn may have a marked influence on the findings reported.

Measurement

Once the sample has been selected, issues arise over measurement (see *Chapter 1*). Are the measures used valid and reliable? Were all the important and relevant characteristics of the individuals measured during the initial data capture? Were all the appropriate outcomes captured during the second phase of data collection? Omissions and failures here can seriously undermine any cohort study. For example, a study that investigated the prognosis for patients with lung disease would need to collect baseline data on smoking habits and environmental exposure to atmospheric irritants. Any failure to do so would leave the findings seriously deficient in terms of their interpretability.

Comparison between groups

Cohort studies are frequently concerned with making comparisons between different subgroups defined by some characteristic at the initial time-point. For example, we might be asking whether smokers fare better or worse than non-smokers in their disease progression; or whether men differ from women in their use of health care resources; or whether those treated on an inpatient basis do better than those seen as outpatients. While such descriptive analyses may be informative, moving from using variables to describe a relationship to using them to explain that relationship can be a slippery slope. Associations between variables do not necessarily indicate that the relationship is causal (*Chapter 7*). The presence of confounding variables can both generate spurious connections and hide real relationships.

A further difficulty in making comparisons occurs when many different subgroups are compared in the search for significant differences. Unless comparisons are relatively few in number and have been pre-specified, such fishing expeditions violate the basic assumptions underlying statistical hypothesis testing (*Chapter 6*).

Follow-up

What differentiates cohort studies from surveys then is the inclusion of a second phase of data collection on the original group of study subjects. As this additional data gathering may take place many months, years or even decades after the first, there is great potential for individuals to get 'lost' to this follow-up. Such losses to follow-up pose important challenges to the validity of cohort study findings. The problem is that those who fall by the wayside are frequently different in important and systematic ways from those who remain in the study. For example, a study that followed up patients after treatment to assess their satisfaction with the services provided might fail to collect data on those who do not keep their clinic appointments. Such losses to follow-up clearly have the potential to bias study findings.

A second problem with follow-up is that sufficient time should have elapsed to allow any phenomena of interest to emerge. Follow-up that is too short may fail to uncover important relationships. A study looking at patient recovery from surgery may miss important chronic discomfort if follow-up is limited to just a few weeks (Macrae and Davies, 1999). The problem with long-term follow-up is that it provides additional opportunities for significant numbers of study subjects to be lost.

Analysis pitfalls

The key analysis of cohort data involves describing patient outcomes at the second time point and relating these to the patients' initial characteristics. There are at least three important ways in which such an analysis can be incomplete or misleading. First, the analysis should take into account any confounding variables and adjust for these. For example, a cohort study that found an apparent relationship between coffee drinking and heart disease would need to adjust the findings for differences between coffee drinkers and non-coffee drinkers in terms of smoking habits, dietary intake and a host of other lifestyle factors. It can be quite difficult to know whether all potential confounders have been adjusted for and this area of the discussion in any published report needs special scrutiny.

A second pitfall in the analysis of cohorts lies in the potential for contemporaneous changes to cloud the findings. One specific instance of this is that patients age as time passes, and therefore any analysis must take account of this. This is only likely to be a problem when the period of follow-up is significantly long. For example, a study that examined the long-term incidence of disease for different occupational groups would need to take into account the fact that many diseases increase with age, and that many occupational groups have different age profiles.

Thirdly, many cohort studies recruit study subjects over a period of time. This then means that there may be different lengths of follow-up on different individuals. This too must be accounted for in the analysis.

Finally, any analysis of cohort data needs to take account of the play of chance (*Chapter 6*). All the measures used to describe the initial cohort can (and should) be presented in terms of both their average and their spread. In addition, the main measures used in cohort analyses (usually relative risks, *Chapter 5*), can all be calculated with confidence intervals. This approach has an important advantage over traditional hypothesis testing in that it presents a range of possible scenarios that are compatible with the empirical data rather than simply denoting statistical significance (Gardner and Altman, 1986).

Retrospective cohorts

We have described cohort studies in terms of the selection and measurement of patients, the elapse of time, and then further data collection on the same group of individuals. Such studies, when carried out in this manner, are called prospective cohorts. There is, however, another way in which cohort studies may be carried out which is conceptually identical but practically advantageous. It concerns an approach to minimise the impact of protracted follow-up. All that waiting around for time to elapse during a cohort study is enough to try anyone's patience, and so an elaboration on the design has evolved. Called **retrospective cohorts**, these studies reach back in to the past to define a cohort at some historical time point. The initial data on this cohort are then collected from historical records of some sort, and subsequent data are gathered either from existing records or through new contacts being made with the individuals. For example, in designing a study relating birth-weight to subsequent intellectual development, we might define a cohort as 'all babies born in a random sample of hospitals in 1971'. Initial data collection would then be captured from old medical records. For the second phase of data collection, sampled individuals could either be traced and interviewed, or school records could be searched to find educational attainment.

The obvious advantage of retrospective cohort studies is the obviation of the need to wait around for time to pass between data collections. Equally obviously, the approach is heavily dependent on the availability, accuracy and completeness of historical data sources. The key pitfalls in retrospective cohort studies are the same as those for prospective studies only writ large: selection bias; measurement deficiencies; and losses to follow-up.

Conclusions

Cohort studies foster an understanding of change in patients, and the relationship of any change with patient and service characteristics. The opportunity to avoid bias and erroneous interpretations makes cohort studies superior to surveys in answering such questions but inferior to randomised controlled trials in assessing cause and effect. Nonetheless, there are many instances when randomised controlled trials are impractical, unethical or otherwise undesirable and thus observational studies like cohort designs have an important role to play (Black, 1996).

Many of the potential biases in survey design are relevant considerations for cohort studies (*Chapter 10*). In addition, further pitfalls lie in inadequate follow-up (in terms of time or completeness), and erroneous analyses (especially lack of attention to confounding factors, including contemporaneous change). More detailed explanations of the design and analysis of cohort studies, and their critical appraisal, can be found in a range of useful texts (Sackett *et al*, 1991; Laupacis *et al*, 1994; Crombie, 1996; Sackett *et al*, 1997).

Key points

* Cohort studies answer questions about what happens to patients over time, and how this experience differs between various patient groups.

* Cohort studies involve two (or more) distinct phases of data collection on the same individuals separated by the passage of time.

* Although data collected in surveys (at a single time point) may be analysed in a longitudinal manner, such analyses are weak and potentially flawed.

* The key areas where bias can creep into cohort studies are: when the patients are selected; when the measures are taken; when patients get lost to follow-up; and when analyses do not properly consider confounding.

* Retrospective cohort studies may be efficient ways of gathering data for long-term studies but they are especially prone to all the main pitfalls found in any cohort design.

References

Black N (1996) Why we need observational studies to evaluate the effectiveness of health care. *Br Med J* **312**: 1215–8
Crombie IK (1996) *The Pocket Guide to Critical Appraisal*. BMJ Publishing, London

Crombie IK, Davies HTO (1998) Selection bias in pain research. *Pain* **74**: 1–3

Gardner MJ, Altman DG (1986) Confidence intervals rather than p-values: estimation rather than hypothesis testing. *Br Med J* **292**: 746–50

Laupacis AG, Wells WS, Richardson, Tugwell P (1994) Users' guides to the medical literature. V. How to use an article about prognosis. *J Am Med Assoc* **272**(3): 234–7

Lieberman BA, Rosenblatt DB, Belsey E *et al* (1979) The effects of maternally administered pethidine or epidural bupivacaine on the fetus and newborn. *Br J Obs Gyn* **86**: 598–606

Macrae WA, Davies HTO (1999) The epidemiology of chronic post-surgical pain. In: Crombie IK, Linton S, Croft P *et al The Epidemiology of Chronic Pain*. International Association for the Study of Pain, Seattle

Sackett DL (1979) Bias in analytical research. *J Chronic Dis* **32**: 51–63

Sackett DL, Haynes RB, Guyatt GH, Tugwell P (1991) *Clinical Epidemiology: A Basic Science for Clinical Medicine*. Little, Brown and Company, Boston, Massachusetts

Sackett DL, Richardson WS, Rosenberg W, Haynes RB (1997) *Evidence-based Medicine: how to practice and teach EBM*. Churchill Livingstone, London

12

Understanding screening

Julian Davis, Iain Crombie, Huw Davies

Screening has generally been successful in identifying those at risk from disease. This success has led to the belief that screening in the general population is always a good thing. However, there are pitfalls which must be avoided if screening programmes are to achieve what is intended for them.

Early physicians would probably have looked with suspicion upon one of their number claiming to be able to identify individuals who have a disease before they showed symptoms; to them it may well have smacked of witchcraft. To us, the advent of modern biochemical and histological techniques has now made this a commonplace fact of clinical life, and a multitude of screening programmes are now in place across the world.

There have been many successful screening programmes, such as that for cervical cancer in the UK. This was initiated in the 1960s, and followed up by the introduction of the national recall system in 1988. This programme has been credited with a reduction in the incidence of cervical cancer of 35% over the fifteen year period up to 1995, and with a significant fall in mortality (Quinn *et al*, 1999).

Screening is usually seen as a good thing, because it uses simple tests to identify disease in a proportion of the population before symptoms present. This can relieve suffering and save lives. As a consequence of this, there is a tendency to call for screening programmes to be set up as soon as a test becomes available. This has been an area of heated debate for many years in both popular and medical journals. For example, the issue of screening for prostate cancer has been a point of contention. Although some articles in the popular press advocate it (Stuttaford, 1995; Smith, 1995), the weight of medical opinion is that its use is not yet justified (Selley *et al*, 1997; Woolf, 1997; Abbasi, 1998). As well as the political drive, there is also a greater direct public interest. Information is now more freely available via the internet, and patients (and potential patients) will discover for themselves the existence and availability of research and of specific tests. The result of this is that the pressure for screening will grow. A positive test can cause great mental distress, and it is important that the requirements for the establishment of a successful and effective screening programme are better and more widely understood.

This chapter aims to give an introduction to the epidemiological basis of screening, to give a brief overview of the ways in which it works (or doesn't), and to highlight some of the problems faced in setting up such programmes.

Why screen, and when is it suitable to do so?

Screening may be defined as the use of testing to identify patients, who have not presented with symptoms, who are at sufficient risk of developing a disorder that it warrants further investigation or treatment. The main aim of screening is to prevent disease, or to minimise its consequences. This may be primary prevention, such as the screening for risk factors for a condition (eg. hypertension in cardiovascular disease), or secondary prevention, such as the early detection of cancer.

Criteria for successful screening

There are a number of criteria which must be satisfied before a screening programme should be launched upon an unsuspecting public. The criteria were set out in depth for the World Health Organization thirty years ago (Wilson and Jungner, 1968). Below is a simplified version of the criteria which are generally accepted attributes of a successful screening test (modified from Mausner and Kramer, 1985).

❖ The condition must be sufficiently common in the target population for the number of cases identified and treated as a result of screening to be significant. A screening programme is complex to establish and maintain, and benefits, in terms of lives saved, must be sufficient to justify this investment.

❖ The condition must have a well-defined latent period, a relatively slow rate of progression from onset, and a well understood natural history. Also, since screening is done on a cyclical basis, the repeat interval for the test should be shorter than the latency of the condition.

❖ There must be a suitable test available for the condition, and the test itself must satisfy certain validity criteria (see below).

❖ There must be an effective (and cost-effective) treatment for the condition — you cannot tell a patient they have a high risk of contracting something if you can do nothing about it. Equally, if a treatment exists, but is not universally available, those screened must be eligible for treatment if it is shown that they are at risk.

❖ The early detection of the condition must substantially improve the prognosis compared to waiting until symptoms present. The margin is clearly a subjective one, but there must be consensus beforehand on what level of improved prognosis is acceptable. There should also be agreement that the proposed screening programme will deliver that improvement.

The screening test itself should not be harmful, frightening, or overly intrusive. Even if a test exists, the take-up (see 'Yield', *p. 106*) will be poor if the test is painful, undignified or unpleasant. For example, sigmoidoscopy screening for rectal cancer is possible, but many patients find the test uncomfortable, and prefer faecal occult blood test screening. This is somewhat less sensitive, but less invasive (Scholefield, 2000). The patient must perceive that taking the test now is much less unpleasant than the threatened symptoms would be several years hence.

The costs must be justified. The costs of screening are considerable, and in today's financial climate, cost-effectiveness is essential. The test itself is often inexpensive, but follow-up testing for positives, treatment if appropriate and all the incidental costs and resources should also be taken into account. Equally, decisions about the basis of recall and patient eligibility can be made with reference to cost-effectiveness (Boer *et al*, 1998). Screening should result in lower costs than treating once symptoms present.

Characteristics of tests

There is no point in initiating a screening programme based upon a test which is not able reliably to detect the condition in which you are interested. There are a number of inherent characteristics which must be assessed when considering if a test is suitable for becoming the basis of a screening programme: **reliability**, **validity** and **yield**.

Reliability

Any screening programme can only be as reliable as the test upon which it is based. A test's reliability depends upon two factors, the test's own repeatability (method variation), and the repeatability with which the results are interpreted (observer variation). The repeatability of the test itself can increasingly be assured by the growing use of technology in the testing process. Observer variation is more difficult to control, since it can not only result from differences between observers, but also from different performances of the same observer at different times. Careful methodology, and intensive training and re-validation can help to reduce these sources of error.

Validity

The validity of a test is a measure of its ability to perform its intended function; that is to detect those in a population who have a given condition, and those who do not. There are two components to validity — sensitivity and specificity. These are inherent characteristics which are vital to the successful use of a test in a screening programme.

Sensitivity

The sensitivity of a test is its accuracy in detecting those individuals in a population who **have** a condition. In mathematical terms, this is the number who **test** positive expressed as a percentage of all those who actually **are** positive, that is to say who have the condition (*Box 12.1*). A test which has a sensitivity of 100% will detect all individuals in a given population who have the condition. It will give no false negatives.

Specificity

The specificity of a test is its ability to identify those individuals who do not have a condition. This is expressed as those who test negative as a percentage of those who are negative (*Box 12.1*). A test with 100% specificity will identify all those who do not have a condition. Such a test will give no false positives.

Box 12.1: How to calculate sensitivity, specificity, positive and negative predictive value

	Disease	No disease
positive test	a	b
negative test	c	d
Total	a+c	b+d

- ❖ Sensitivity = a/ (a+c) x 100
- ❖ Specificity = d/ (b+d) x 100
- ❖ Positive predictive value = a/ (a+b) x 100
- ❖ Negative predictive value = d/ (c+d) x 100

The sensitivity/specificity trade-off

The majority of tests do not have 100% sensitivity and specificity. In other words they are generally better either at identifying sufferers or non-sufferers, but not both. As with much in life, the result is a trade-off, in which the decision must be made as to where to draw the line between two extremes.

A simple example will serve to illustrate this point. The hypothetical data in *Table 12.1* show a sample of patients who are to be part of a screening exercise for kidney disease. The test used is the serum creatinine level.

The trade-off is illustrated by *Table 12.2*, in which the sensitivity and specificity are calculated by using the numbers from *Table 12.1* and the formula from *Box 12.1*. As the cut-off point is moved, so the balance between specificity and sensitivity changes. If the choice is made to classify all patients with a blood creatinine of >100 mg/100ml as having kidney disease, the sensitivity is excellent as the test will pick up all patients who have kidney disease. However, the specificity is poor, and this means that the test will also pick up a great many patients with normal renal function — false positives.

At the other extreme, if the cut-off is set at 180mg/100ml, the specificity increases, reducing the number of false positives dramatically, but the sensitivity suffers, leaving 10 patients who do have kidney disease undetected — false negatives.

A cut-off of 140mg/100ml gives a compromise in which both sensitivity and specificity are over 80%. Clearly this cut-off point can be moved to suit the primary purpose of the screening test, whether this is identification of those at risk, or reassurance of those who are not.

Table 12.1: The sensitivity/specificity trade-off

Serum creatinine (mg/100ml)	<100	100–139	140–179	180–199	≥200	Total
Patients with normal kidney function	41	152	32	2	0	227
Patients with kidney disease	0	4	6	9	15	34

Table 12.2: Moving the cut-off point

Serum creatinine cut-off	Test sensitivity	Test specificity
≥100	100%	18.1%
≥140	88.2%	85.0%
≥180	70.6%	99.1%
≥200	44.1%	100%

The effect of prevalence

The sensitivity and specificity are not in themselves sufficient to predict whether a given test will perform well in identifying a particular individual with a given condition. The prevalence of the condition in the population is also an important factor.

Again, in order to explain this, we will use a fictitious example. Suppose we have developed a test that has a sensitivity of 95%, and a specificity of 90%, for detecting a mythical condition. We are interested in a sample of 1500 patients who may have this condition. However, if we select our samples from different populations, the results will be very different.

Testing in the outpatient clinic

In the first scenario, the sample is drawn from those attending a hospital outpatient clinic. Here, patients are more likely to be suffering from disease, since they will have been referred there on the basis of symptoms. For this example, assume the prevalence of our condition in this population is 20%. *Table 12.3* illustrates how the numbers work out.

Table 12.3: Fictitious data for illustration of the prevalence problem. Scenario I — in the outpatient clinic

	Disease sensitivity 95%	No disease specificity 90%	Total
positive test	285	120	405
negative test	15	1080	1095
Total	300	1200	1500

Positive predictive value = 70.4%; negative predictive value = 98.6%

Before testing, we know that each individual has a 20% chance of having the disease and an 80% chance of not having it (we can tell this from the prevalence). After testing, the positive and negative predictive values update these figures according to whether the test was positive or negative. If the test is positive, the chance of actually having the disease is now seen to be 70%; if the test is negative the chance of not having the disease is now 98.6%. So, whatever the test result we now know much more than we did before.

Testing in the community

In the second scenario, the sample is drawn instead from the community. Here, the prevalence of our hypothetical condition is only 2%. *Table 12.4* shows what effect this has on the positive and negative predictive values. Although a negative test is now almost definitive (99.9% sure that there really is no disease), a positive test only gives a 16.5% chance of there really being a disease. Because of the lower initial prevalence in the community compared to the clinic, the test performs much less well — and erroneously identifies many well people as sick.

The message from this is that the prevalence of a condition has a powerful effect on the ability of a screening test to identify which patients are at risk. If a screening programme is to be instigated in a particular setting, it is important to know beforehand that the prevalence of the condition in that population is sufficiently high to allow the test to identify correctly a high proportion of sufferers.

Table 12.4: Fictitious data for illustration of the prevalence problem. Scenario 2 — in the community			
	Disease sensitivity 95%	No disease specificity 90%	Total
positive test	29	147	176
negative test	1	1323	1324
Total	30	1470	1500

Positive predictive value = 16.5%; negative predictive value = 99.9%

Yield

The number of previously undiagnosed cases of disease which are picked up by a screening programme is the yield. This is obviously affected by the test itself, and by the prevalence of the condition. However, it is also affected by the frequency with which the test is applied (the recall period) and by the proportion of the population who take up the opportunity to be screened (Jepson *et al*, 2000). Screening programmes need to be 'sold' to the population to encourage take-up, and tests which are invasive or painful are less likely to be popular! A recent development is the concept of the 'number needed to screen' (Rembold, 1998) which formalises the means of deciding how many people should be screened for how long in order to prevent one death.

The future

The number of screening programmes will continue to increase. Technological advance will provide new and more accurate tests for conditions of all kinds, and as intimated earlier, this will drive demand for screening. It is important that the potential pitfalls of screening are not overlooked, and that the ability to detect disease is not allowed to outstrip the ability to treat it. If screening programmes are established before there is consensus within the medical community on their effectiveness, the public will receive conflicting messages, and uptake will suffer. Above all, if the prime tenet of screening — don't screen unless you can treat — is violated, the credibility of screening as a tool in medicine will be severely undermined. If this happens, it will be a long and hard job to re-establish public confidence.

Key points

* Screening has been very successful at reducing the consequences of disease.

* Screening is often assumed to be universally good — this is not always true.

* There are a number of criteria which must be satisfied before a screening programme becomes viable.

* The test itself must have certain attributes which define its effectiveness.

* Screening will become more common, and care must be taken not to allow quality to suffer at the expense of quantity.

References

Abbasi K (1998) To screen or not to screen? *Br Med J* **316**: 484

Boer R, de Koning H, Threlfall A (1998) Cost effectiveness of shortening screening interval or extending age range of NHS breast screening programme: computer simulation study. *Br Med J* **317**: 376

Jepson R, Clegg A, Forbes C (2000) The determinants of screening uptake and interventions for increasing uptake: a systematic review. *Health Technol Assess* **4**(14)

Mausner J, Kramer S (1985) *Epidemiology, an introductory text*. WB Saunders, Philadelphia

Quinn M, Babb P, Jones J (1999) Effect of screening on incidence of and mortality from cancer of the cervix in England: evaluation based on routinely collected statistics. *Br Med J* **318**: 904–908

Rembold C (1998) Number needed to screen: development of a statistic for disease screening. *Br Med J* **317**: 307

Scholefield J (2000) Screening (ABC of colorectal cancer). *Br Med J* **321**: 1004

Selley S, Donovan J, Faulkner A (1997) Diagnosis, management and screening of early localised prostate cancer. *Health Technol Assess* **1**(2)

Smith R (1995) Conflict of interest in The Times. *Br Med J* **310**: 1417

Stuttaford T (1995) Plain guide to the health checks every man and woman needs each year. *The Times*: 16 May

Wilson J, Jungner F (1968) *Pubic Health Papers No 34: Principles and Practice of screening for disease*. World Health Organization, Geneva

Woolf S (1997) Should we screen for prostate cancer? *Br Med J* **314**: 989

13

Bias in case-control studies

Huw Davies, Iain Crombie

Case-control studies are largely used to explore differences between groups of individuals. They can identify potential risk factors associated with disease, or they can investigate patient behaviour, such as why some people do not attend for services. As such, case-control studies are often used to generate or test hypotheses about causal factors. Nonetheless, bias is always a danger in case-control studies, arising especially from the way in which study samples are selected or from the collection of retrospective data. Confounding too remains a problem. This chapter explores ways in which such flaws can be uncovered in published studies.

Epidemiology is concerned with identifying and assessing causal factors related to disease; clinical epidemiology in turn addresses the amelioration of that disease as a result of interventions. Both branches of study use a variety of research designs to uncover these causal relationships between patient characteristics, experiences and health service interventions on the one hand, and health outcomes on the other. Randomised controlled trials offer the strongest evidence of cause and effect (*Chapter 14*), but in many circumstances they can be unethical or impractical. Cohort studies, as discussed previously (*Chapter 11*), can also help unravel what happens to patients and why, but again problems in execution and interpretation abound (*Chapters 11* and *7*).

There are many reasons why prospective studies such as trials or cohort studies might be impractical, inappropriate or unethical. For example, assessing the damaging effects of exposure to various pathogens clearly cannot be countenanced as an experimental design — one cannot imagine randomly allocating patients to smoke 20 cigarettes a day. Even passive observation of potentially harmful exposures poses serious ethical dilemmas. In addition, long-term or very rare outcomes may be impractical to study using prospective designs. In such situations case-control studies offer some advantages. They are relatively cheap and, because they focus on events that have already occurred, relatively quick to conduct. In addition, they can assess the importance of a wide range of possible causative factors in a single study.

The essence of case-control studies is simple. A group of 'cases' are selected — usually individuals with a specific disease — and these cases are then compared to a group who do not have the disease or other defining characteristic of the cases (these are the controls). Differences between the two groups are then explored in an attempt to 'explain' how cases get to be cases. Thus case-control studies are retrospective, looking backwards from a condition to its antecedents. This is in fundamental contrast to trials and cohort studies, which move forwards from exposure to outcomes.

Most often, case-control studies are used to explore disease aetiology or the harmful impacts of various exposures or lifestyles. More rarely they have sometimes been used to examine the long-term benefits of interventions such as screening or vaccination. In principle, case-control studies can be used to explore what it is that makes any group different from another — whether the groups are defined by disease status or by some other marker.

For all the basic simplicity of design, case-control studies are rather prone to bias, perhaps even more so than other observational studies such as cohort designs. Bias can arise in three different areas: in the ways in which both cases and controls are selected; in the ways in which measures are taken; and in the potential for confounding. This chapter explores these biases and advises on their identification and assessment.

The right design

The first issue when confronted with a published report of a case-control study is to ask whether the approach used is the most appropriate. For example, would a prospective cohort study be practical and offer better information? Often the answer to this is 'no' — especially when the outcomes examined are rare, long-term or unexpected. In such cases, a case-control study may be the best that can be expected. However, if the issue under examination can be studied by other means, then the findings from case-control studies should be regarded as preliminary — more hypothesis raising than definitive findings.

Sample selection

The individuals included in a case-control study consist of two separate groups: the cases and the controls. Selection of each poses distinct problems. First, there is the problem of defining 'caseness': what is it that makes a case a case? Often, when examining disease aetiology, a case is defined by some diagnostic criteria. In other studies different characteristics will be used, for example, 'non-attenders' in studies examining why people miss appointments, or 'employment status' in studies examining the factors associated with career success. The crucial issue is that the definitions should be clear-cut and consistently applied: random mis-classification errors in the cases can dilute possible findings, whereas systematic mis-classification errors can lead to specious results.

The second problem in selecting cases is the need for these to be in some senses 'typical'. If the cases selected are highly atypical then any associations discovered may not generalise — limiting the usefulness of the research. For example, cases selected from tertiary referral centres may differ in important ways from those with the same disease seen in general practice.

Cases are only one half of a case-control study, and it is in the selection of controls that the biggest potential pitfalls lie. For comparisons to have any validity, the controls need to be as similar as possible to the cases — excepting, of course, that controls should lack the defining features of 'caseness'. Because cases and controls are selected separately from potentially very different populations, the concern is that it is these selection forces which may account for any differences found between the two groups — leading to spurious findings. The crucial question to ask of the controls used is: how might these controls differ in important ways from the cases because of the way in which they were selected?

In order to get a better match between cases and controls it is not unusual for studies to 'match' controls to pre-existing cases on a number of different criteria (age, sex etc). While this approach may lead to similar looking groups it does complicate the analysis, which should now take account of this matching process.

Measurement

Measurement bias poses a serious problem for almost every research study (*Chapter 1*). In case-control studies, the first challenge is to the integrity of the cases themselves. Measurement errors may, for example, cause non-cases to be identified as cases, or *vice versa*. The first point of scrutiny for measurement errors should be the case definition criteria.

Beyond sample identification, the key role of measurement is to explore possible antecedent factors in both groups. Clearly, to maintain comparability, identical data gathering strategies should be used for both groups. A useful methodological safeguard in this process is 'blinding' of the data gatherers — so that they do not know whether they are collating data for cases or controls. This prevents differential assessments creeping in to the data set.

It is, however, in the retrospective nature of cohort studies that some of the biggest measurement difficulties lie. Study subjects will only rarely be 'blind' to the nature of their condition, and this self-knowledge may impact severely on recollections or assessments of the past. For example, close questioning of parents who have suffered a cot death (the cases) may cause much greater revelation of otherwise minor events (such as mild illness) than would similar questioning of non-bereaved parents (the controls). Whatever the care taken to ensure comparability, recall bias may undermine even well executed case-control studies.

Analysis issues

Case-control studies do not usually draw their cases or their controls from a known population — and therefore cannot provide either incidence or prevalence figures. Unlike cohort studies (*Chapter 11*), it is not possible to calculate relative risks. Instead, the standard measure of comparison is the odds ratio (*Chapter 5*). This measure is in fact a reasonably good estimate of the relative risk for a wide range of circumstances (Davies *et al*, 1998).

The unadjusted odds ratio provides only the first look at associations between antecedent factors and caseness. Although controls may have been selected to try to ensure compatibility with the cases there may be many reasons to suspect that they are different. The possibility of confounding remains a real possibility (*Chapter 7*). Adjusting for a wide range of possible confounders produces a new set of adjusted odds ratios which try to take any known confounders into account. Of course, the possibility that there are significant unknown confounders can never be entirely discounted.

Any case-control analysis needs to take account of the play of chance (see Brennan and Croft, 1994; and *Chapter 6*). The main measures used in the analyses (usually adjusted and unadjusted odds ratios) should all be presented with confidence intervals. This approach has an important advantage over traditional hypothesis testing in that it presents a range of possible scenarios that are compatible with the empirical data rather than simply denoting statistical significance (Gardner and Altman, 1986). This allows the reader to assess both worse-case and best-case scenarios compatible with the data, thus protecting against over-interpretation. In particular, wide confidence intervals around the odds ratio denote studies which have little power to detect even sizeable real effects.

Finally, one of the strengths of the case-control study — its ability to explore a wide range of possible aetiological factors in a single study — also presents some serious dangers when it comes to statistical analysis. The basic premises of hypothesis testing mean that one comparison in 20 will appear as 'statistically significant' by chance alone. Studies which make many comparisons will inevitably 'discover' some spurious results. This is another reason why the findings from case-control studies should be seen as provisional, unless the study was driven by a limited number of prior hypotheses and the analysis was confined to these factors.

Conclusions

Case-control studies sometimes suffer from serious biases that may be difficult to avoid or even quantify. The title of a review in this area (A collection of 56 topics with contradictory results in case-control studies [Mayes *et al*, 1988]) attests to the potentially misleading nature of the design. Nonetheless, case-control studies do have a role to play in exploring factors associated with rare, unexpected or long-term events. They also provide a valuable service in raising hypotheses that may subsequently be investigated using more robust methods.

The key sources of bias in case-control studies arise from the ways in which samples are selected and measurements are taken. Atypical cases may limit the conclusions that can be drawn from studies, and carelessly drawn controls can vitiate any comparisons. The unavoidably retrospective nature of the design places important limits on the quality of the data that can be gathered and always raises the spectre of recall bias. As with all observational designs the possibility of confounding can never be entirely excluded when interpreting any associations found.

More detailed explanations of the design and analysis of case-control studies can be found in a range of useful texts (Schlesselman, 1982; Sackett *et al*, 1991; Levine, *et al*, 1994; Crombie, 1996; Sackett *et al*, 1997). Some of these provide handy checklists for critical appraisal of the design.

Key points

* Case-control studies try to answer questions about why individuals with some defining characteristic (often a disease; the cases) differ from individuals without that characteristic (the controls).

* Case-control studies are unavoidably retrospective in nature, moving from some outcome to explore a range of antecedent factors. The quality of evidence they produce is usually considered inferior to that arising from prospective studies.

* Case-control studies may be most appropriate for the investigation of rare, long-term or unexpected outcomes, or for exploring a range of novel aetiological hypotheses.

* Bias in case-control studies arises primarily from the ways in which samples are selected (especially in the choosing of appropriate controls), and from the ways in which data are collected (especially because of the possibility of recall bias).

* Good case-control studies are tentative in their conclusions and feature the following key attributes: clear and reliable definitions of 'caseness'; identical identification and data gathering procedures for controls; an assessment of the potential impact of recall bias; and a comprehensive exploration of the possibility of confounding.

References

Brennan P, Croft P (1994) Interpreting the results of observational research: chance is not such a fine thing. *Br Med J* **309**: 727–30

Crombie IK (1996) *The Pocket Guide to Critical Appraisal*. BMJ Publishing, London

Davies HTO, Crombie IK, Tavakoli M (1998) When can odds ratios mislead? *Br Med J* **316**: 689–91

Gardner MJ, Altman DG (1986) Confidence intervals rather than p-values: estimation rather than hypothesis testing. *Br Med J* **292**: 746–50

Levine M, Walter S *et al* (1994) Users' guides to the medical literature. IV. How to use an article about harm. *J Am Med Assoc* **271**(20): 1615–19

Mayes LC, Horwitz RI *et al* (1988) A collection of 56 topics with contradictory results in case-control research. *Int J Epidemiol* **17**(3): 680–5

Sackett DL, Haynes RB *et al* (1991) *Clinical Epidemiology: A Basic Science for Clinical Medicine*. Little, Brown and Company, Boston, Massachusetts

Sackett DL, Richardson WS *et al* (1997) *Evidence-based Medicine: how to practice and teach EBM*. Churchill Livingstone, London

Schlesselman JJ (1982) *Case-Control Studies: Design, Conduct, Analysis*. Oxford University Press, New York

14

Bias in treatment trials

Huw Davies

Rigorous treatment trials exhibit a number of key features to guard against bias. Randomisation, blinding (of patients, care staff and assessors), full follow-up on all patients, and 'intention-to-treat' analyses all contribute to removing bias so that any true treatment effect can be revealed. This chapter outlines the rationale behind these features and advises how bias in treatment trials can be assessed.

Clinicians, health care managers and even policy makers are increasingly questioning the effectiveness of health care interventions. At the same time, a growing reservoir of research evidence provides some guidance. However not all research evidence on the effectiveness of treatments is a reliable guide: treatment trials can be flawed in design, execution or analysis. This chapter outlines the key areas where bias may arise in treatment trials. It is in these areas that discerning readers will search for problems when appraising the quality of research evidence.

Why carry out randomised control trials?

Personal experience provides a poor guide for physicians when it comes to assessing the effectiveness of treatment interventions (Crombie and Davies, 1996; Davies and Nutley, 1999). Patients get better by themselves, often despite, not because of interventions. The placebo effect (benefits arising which are non-specific to the therapy) and the clouding effects of chance variability also conspire to obscure any true estimate of treatment effect. History has shown that treatment studies without appropriate controls are apt to mislead (Gilbert *et al*, 1977; Pocock, 1983). Historical controls (comparing current treatment success with previous patient outcomes), and concurrent non-randomised controls (comparing new treatments with existing practice but with no experimental allocation of patients between these two groups), both prove susceptible to bias. Control groups need to be concurrent and randomly assigned.

117

The importance of concealed randomisation

Random allocation of patients to either the new treatment under test or some comparative therapy is the cornerstone of a good quality trial. Such random allocation provides no guarantees. However, given sufficient patient numbers, randomisation makes it likely that the two groups will be evenly matched — both for factors known to be important in determining outcome (age, severity etc) and also for those factors whose prognostic value may be unknown but nonetheless crucial (for example, genetic makeup). It is randomisation that leads (on average) to balanced groups and fair comparisons.

Randomisation can be achieved in a number of different ways. For example, envelopes containing group allocation may be provided in advance, or clinicians recruiting new patients may telephone a central co-ordinator to learn the group allocation of the next patient. Some methods of randomisation are more secure than others; that is, they are less prone to manipulation by clinicians who favour one treatment avenue over another. There is some evidence that randomisation that is not tamper proof may not be immune from bias (Schulz *et al*, 1995). In appraising the quality of a trial, it may be worth asking not only was the allocation to new treatment and control carried out randomly, but also was the random allocation secure from interference or prediction.

Checking for equivalence at baseline

Random allocation of patients to 'new treatment' and 'control' groups will on average lead to fair and balanced groups. This tendency increases as the number of patients increases. However, it is possible that, even when the randomisation was well conducted, just by chance, the two groups may not be as evenly balanced as hoped. In analysing trial data, it is usual to first of all compare and present the composition of the two groups 'at baseline' (ie. just after randomisation and before treatments have been applied). This comparison seeks reassurance that the two groups are indeed similar on all known patient variables. Any significant differences found between the two groups may need to be taken into consideration when assessing the treatment outcomes.

The importance of blinding

The key features of rigorous trials after randomisation try to ensure that both groups are handled identically thereafter to prevent any imbalances creeping in. A key tool here is blinding.

'Single blinding' is achieved when patients are unaware of whether they are receiving the new treatment under test or the control treatment. This protects against the placebo effect and patient mis-report arising from differential expectations about the likely impact of treatment. Of course, such concealment should also extend to those assessing the treatment outcomes, otherwise knowledge of which treatment group patients are in may bias the assessor's judgement (Noseworthy *et al*, 1994).

'Double blinding' is achieved when not only are the patients unaware of their treatment group, but so are their physicians and other care staff. This approach guards against patients being treated differently because of knowledge about their group allocation. Good studies often try to conceal group allocation even during the final analysis (sometimes called 'triple blinding') to prevent any bias creeping in during data analysis and interpretation.

Although blinding in all its forms is an essential bulwark against bias it may be difficult or impossible to achieve (eg. in trials of physical therapies or surgery, [Deyo *et al*, 1990]). Even when possible, blinding may be incomplete, for example, patients may be able to tell which group they are in because of the distinctive characteristics of new and old treatments. Presentation of some data on the success or otherwise of blinding (among both patients and staff) may help to clarify the potential for bias.

Identifying a clear study population

The reader of any treatment trial needs to know about the patients studied so that they can decide whether or not the findings are applicable to other patient populations. Reports of treatment studies should provide a clear description not only of the patients included in the study but also how they were drawn. That is, they should describe the planned study population, the sites where individuals were recruited into the study, the inclusion or exclusion criteria that were used to signify suitability for the trial, and the number of rejections or refusals. This kind of information is best presented as a flow chart (JAMA Instructions for Authors, *JAMA* 1998, **279**: 71). Close inspection of these numbers allows the reader to determine whether or not the patients studied are likely to be 'typical' and the implications this has for interpretation of any treatment effect found. This form of presentation will also help account for any lost patients or transfers between the two treatment groups — both of which have implications for the assessment of bias.

Checking for full patient follow-up and 'intention-to-treat analysis'

Randomisation helps lead to balanced groups at baseline. What happens to group composition after this can compromise any balance and lead to unfair comparisons. First, patients lost to follow-up after they have been allocated to groups give cause for concern. Even if similar numbers of patients are lost from each treatment group, the worry is that different sorts of patients may be being lost. Suppose, for example, that patients with the more severe disease drop out from one group and those with milder disease drop out from the other. This would lead to imbalances between the groups and would bias the findings. Similarly, concerns arise over patients who swap between treatment groups, ie. those patients who, for whatever reason, sub- sequently receive care different from that originally allocated to them.

Because of these concerns about the balance between groups being upset, the key analysis should compare the groups as originally allocated. This is called an 'intention-to-treat analysis'. Such an analysis is the simplest way to prevent bias creeping in from differential loss of patients or differential movement between treatment groups. If no data on treatment outcomes are available for some patients, then an analysis that assumes that these outcomes were poor can help clarify whether or not the overall findings are susceptible to bias from these losses.

'Intention-to-treat analyses' answer a very precise question. They are not trying to answer the question:

> *Does treatment A produce better*
> *outcomes than treatment B?*

Instead, they address the much more pragmatic issue of:

> *Does a decision to use treatment A produce better*
> *outcomes on aggregate than a decision to use treatment*
> *B (even if that decision cannot always be seen through*
> *to completion)?*

Intention-to-treat analyses help avoid bias and answer pragmatic questions of real interest to clinicians faced with making treatment choices.

Coping with the clouding effects of chance

Preventing bias does not guarantee that trials will always reveal any real underlying treatment effects. Chance variability can conspire to mislead in even the best-planned clinical trials. *Figure 14.1* shows how, just through chance, the findings from any single trial may mismatch the true situation. Trials may mislead in two ways: they may show an apparent effect which is not real; or they may appear to show no difference when in fact one treatment is truly superior in effect.

		Real situation:	
		No worthwhile difference between new and old treatment	*Worthwhile difference between new and old treatment*
What the study finds:	*No statistical difference between new and old treatment*	Study correctly matches true situation	**Misleading result:** Can happen by chance. Power calculation tells how often. (Type II error)
	Statistically significant difference between new and old treatment	**Misleading result:** Can happen by chance. Significance level tells how often. (Type I error)	Study correctly matches true situation.

Figure 14.1: Possible matches and mismatches between 'truth' and study findings brought about by chance

Detailed guidance on assessing the impact of chance in treatment trials has been given elsewhere (*Chapter 6*). In brief, it is the statistical significance level that tells of the likelihood of making the first error, and it is the power calculation that provides information on the likelihood of the second. There is always a trade-off between these two errors: as we try to avoid one we become more likely to commit the other. The only way out of this bind is an increase in sample size.

A further complication lies in the question 'when is a difference a worthwhile difference?' This is a question about clinical, as compared to statistical, significance. We cannot easily assess how likely we are to be led astray by chance until we have answered that question. Looking for small effects is more demanding than searching for large differences. What is more, chance variability can only be assessed once bias has been dismissed as a major factor in the findings (Brennan and Croft, 1994). A number of useful sources provide further elaboration of the tricky issues surrounding sample size, power and the assessment of the play of chance (Altman and Bland, 1995; Eypasch *et al*, 1995; Florey, 1993; Gardner and Altman, 1986).

Pre-specification of relevant outcomes and subgroup analyses

Statistical considerations also impact on the range of variables that can be explored for differences in clinical trials. Good clinical trials specify in advance the key outcome of interest. This outcome is then the primary focus of the analysis (it is usually termed 'the primary endpoint'). This pre-specification is necessary because otherwise the basis for the statistical tests used to distinguish potentially real effects from likely chance differences is undermined. The very definition of statistical significance means that for every 20 variables examined one is likely to show a 'statistically significant difference' by chance alone, even when there is no true difference. It is for the same reason that subgroup analyses should always be specified in advance — and be limited to few comparisons with some underlying biological plausibility. Again, comparing many different subgroups in an *ad hoc* manner is likely to lead to spurious findings.

Concluding remarks

This chapter has focused on highlighting those areas to examine when going in search of bias in treatment trials. Many other equally important issues arise when examining reports of clinical trials. Most of these have been covered in previous chapters and they are not examined in detail here:

❖ Were the treatments under study the most appropriate to compare? The treatment given to controls should be the next best alternative to the treatment under study. Comparing new therapies to 'no intervention' or 'placebo' is only appropriate when no suitable comparison treatment exists.

❖ Were the treatments under study well defined and clearly described? Were they delivered in readily replicable settings?

❖ Are the benefits, such as they might be, worth the costs (*Chapters 8* and *9*)? Were all the possible benefits enumerated and assessed (*Chapter 8*)? What about issues of safety (Eypasch *et al*, 1995)? Were patient preferences incorporated (*Chapter 17*)? Were the benefits portrayed in both absolute and relative terms (*Chapter 5*)?

Assessment of bias must take place before any statistical judgements on the effects can be made (Brennan and Croft 1994). A number of places in the design, execution and analysis of trials need careful inspection: randomisation and its tamper-proof nature; blinding and the success of concealment achieved in practice; the completeness of follow-up and the use of an 'intention-to-treat' analysis; the appropriate handling of chance variability with a clear declaration of the power of the study to uncover real and worthwhile effects. Further guidance on these issues is available from a number of published sources and checklists in this area (Crombie, 1996; Guyatt *et al*, 1993; Guyatt *et al*, 1994; Sackett *et al*, 1997).

Finally, individual treatment trials should not be viewed in isolation. As more and better quality systematic reviews and meta-analyses are becoming available, single trials need to be interpreted in the context of this wider body of information (*Chapter 15*).

Key points

* The key objective in any treatment trial is for fair comparisons.

* Initial balance between treatment groups is best achieved by random allocation between new and old treatments. Randomisation should be properly concealed to avoid manipulation.

* Treatment groups should be assessed for their equivalence at baseline as randomisation does not guarantee balance.

* Ensuring fair comparison thereafter depends on blinding all participants (patients, health care staff, assessors and even analysts) to the individual patient's group allocation.

* The success of the blinding should be assessed to investigate possible sources of bias.

* As far as possible, all patients should be followed up, and an 'intention-to-treat analysis' on the primary endpoint should be performed. Subgroup analyses need to be treated with circumspection.

* Chance variability can mislead by creating spurious effects or hiding real ones. Before chance effects can be estimated, bias must be ruled out.

References

Altman DG, Bland JM (1995) Absence of evidence is not evidence of absence. *Br Med J* **311**: 485

Brennan P, Croft P (1994) Interpreting the results of observational research: chance is not such a fine thing. *Br Med J* **309**: 727–30

Crombie IK (1996) *The Pocket Guide to Critical Appraisal.* BMJ Publishing, London

Crombie IK, Davies HTO (1996) *Research in Health Care: design conduct and interpretation of health services research.* John Wiley & Sons, Chichester

Davies HTO, Nutley SM (1999) The rise and rise of evidence in health care. *Public Money Manage* **19**: 9–16

Deyo RA, Walsh NE, Schoenfeld LS, Ramamurthy S (1990) Can trials of physical treatments be blinded? The example of transcutaneous electrical nerve stimulation for chronic pain. *Am J Phys Med Rehab* **69**: 6–10

Eypasch E, Lefering R, Kum CK, Troidl H (1995) Probability of adverse events that have not yet occurred: a statistical reminder. *Br Med J* **311**: 619–20

Florey CV (1993) Sample size for beginners. *Br Med J* **306**:1181–4

Gardner MJ, Altman DG (1986) Confidence intervals rather than p-values: estimation rather than hypothesis testing. *Br Med J* **292**: 746–50

Gilbert JP, McPeek B, Mosteller F (1977) Statistics and ethics in surgery and anesthesia. *Science* **198**: 684–9

Guyatt GH, Sackett DL, Cook DJ (1993) Users' guides to the medical literature. II. How to use an article about therapy or prevention. A. Are the results of the study valid? *J Am Med Assoc* **270**: 2598–601

Guyatt GH, Sackett DL, Cook DJ (1994) Users' guides to the medical literature. II. How to use an article about therapy or prevention. B. What were the results and will they help me in caring for my patients? *J Am Med Assoc* **271**: 59–63

Noseworthy JH, Ebers GC, Vandervoort MK, Farquhar RE, Yetisir E, Roberts R (1994) The impact of blinding on the results of a randomized, placebo-controlled multiple sclerosis clinical trial. *Neurology* **44**: 16–20

Pocock SJ (1983) *Clinical Trials: A Practical Approach.* John Wiley & Sons, Chichester

Sackett DL, Richardson WS, Rosenberg W, Haynes RB (1997) *Evidence-based Medicine: how to practice and teach EBM.* Churchill Livingstone, London

Schulz K, Chalmers I, Hayes RJ, Altman DG (1995) Empirical evidence of bias: dimensions of methodological quality associated with estimates of treatment effects in controlled trials. *J Am Med Assoc* **273**: 408–12

15

Getting to grips with systematic reviews and meta-analyses

Huw Davies, Iain Crombie

Systematic reviews and meta-analyses now form a major source of evidence on clinical effectiveness. Despite the relative recency of this approach to synthesising research findings, a reasonable consensus has emerged as to the desirable methodological characteristics of this secondary research. Understanding these basic tenets enables readers to take a balanced view of published review findings.

The past decade has seen an unprecedented interest in evidence of clinical effectiveness. Health care professionals, managers and policy makers are looking more than ever before to the evidence-base in support of decision-making. In tandem with this growing interest, there has been an explosion of activity aimed at synthesising and exploiting the expanding research literature. At the forefront of this activity has been the development of approaches to research synthesis and review which are rigorous and unbiased. Understanding the new methodologies of systematic review and meta-analysis, and learning to tell rigorous from non-rigorous review, is becoming an essential skill for those who wish to develop more evidence-based care.

Why review?

Clinical trials aim to distinguish effective therapies from the harmful or the useless. Yet in any given therapeutic area there may be many primary research studies examining the effectiveness of specific interventions — sometimes far too many for any individual practitioner to read them all. Hence the need for review papers. When many studies do exist it is not unusual for some to be inconclusive (unable to demonstrate benefits, but unable to exclude the possibility either), or for others to be in conflict (some studies appearing to show benefit while others do not). The problem for the decision maker lies in making sense of a literature which may be large, diverse and dispersed.

Making sense of a contradictory mass of evidence was for a long time the domain of the clinical expert as review writer. Many different styles of article purport to review important therapeutic questions: overviews, editorials, commentaries, consensus statements or guidelines may all fall into this category. However, in the late 1980s Cynthia Mulrow drew attention to the comparative lack of rigour in secondary research (where the unit of study is other research studies) compared to primary research (studies involving fresh data collection [Mulrow, 1987]). She concluded that in many reviews the conclusions stated are not justified by the available evidence. As David Sackett and colleagues said in their text 'Clinical Epidemiology', 'we think that the reason for this deficiency... lies in the tradition of calling upon content-area experts... these authors begin their task with a conclusion... little wonder, then, that the results may be skewed in content and citation as well as conclusion' (Sackett *et al*, 1991). Whatever the reasons, the message is clear: narrative reviews are frequently misleading. The response to this exposure of the traditional narrative review process as flawed was the development of a new rigorous tradition: systematic reviews.

In this way it was hoped that the advantages of reviews could be maintained and misleading conclusions could be minimised. The advantages lie in the greater power provided by aggregating data from a complete set of studies. This brings with it a diminution of the play of chance and allows the emergence of a clearer picture and a more precise estimate of any treatment effect. Thus new knowledge may be extracted from existing studies which are not individually all that informative.

The essence of unbiased review

The desirable requirements of an unbiased review are simple in conception but rather harder to obtain in practice. The starting point is a complete list of all relevant studies. Deciding whether a study is relevant is often no easy matter. First, it should be addressing the appropriate research question, and second it should itself have been carried out with methodological rigour. Ensuring that the list is complete is troublesome and the concern is that studies missed in the review may tell a different story than those included. Once a suitable set of original studies has been amassed, the difficulty lies in aggregating the data across the studies (giving each study its due weight) in order to estimate an overall effect size. This new information is then interpreted in the light of the diversity of studies included in the review. At each stage of the review the intention is to ensure that decisions taken are first, as far as possible, unbiased, and second that they are well documented and open to scrutiny.

Pitfalls in reviews

Despite the rigorous methodology by which systematic reviews should be conducted (Cook *et al,* 1995) problems can still arise. As with primary research, flaws may creep into reviews during any of the major stages of design, execution or interpretation. To assist the reader to uncover deficiencies in published work, the issues relating to these pitfalls are discussed in more detail.

Inappropriate review questions

Good review questions are expressed with clarity and focus. Each of four main dimensions needs to be specified:

- the intervention of interest
- the patient groups to whom the intervention is applied
- the primary outcome(s) which the intervention is intended to promote or avert
- the settings (including aspects of concomitant care) in which the intervention is applied.

Lack of clarity or specificity in any of these areas may diminish (but not necessarily demolish) interest or confidence in the findings.

Inadequate identification of original studies

The starting point for any review is a complete (as possible) collection of relevant studies. A complete set of studies is achieved by thorough searching, not just of the most convenient electronic sources such as Medline, but including more elusive published reports, such as those in conference proceedings, and hard-to-get-at unpublished sources, such as industry trials (the so-called 'grey literature'). The best reviewers may even resort to hand searching of journals, personal requests to known investigators and even trawling of funding bodies' archives. They will also not confine the review to English-language reports, but will examine the international literature.

In gathering together a set of studies for a review the key concern is one of selection bias: is there any way in which the studies included might be systematically different from those that have been missed? In truth, there are many ways in which this can happen:

> *Studies with significant results are more likely to get published than studies without significant results,... those with significant results are more likely to get published in English, more likely to be cited and more likely to be published repeatedly,... [and] may be more likely to get published in a journal indexed in a literature database.*

Egger and Davey-Smith, 1998

To overcome these difficulties, good reviews will first of all be as thorough as possible in searching for relevant studies, and secondly they will describe in detail the search strategy used and the criteria employed in gathering primary studies. In this way readers of the review can judge for themselves the appropriateness of the initial studies uncovered.

Inappropriate selection of studies

Not all studies uncovered will be suitable for inclusion in the review: some will be more relevant than others. The relevance of any individual study is defined first by the topic it addresses and second by the quality of its methodology. The preliminary search might, for example, uncover primary studies which are insufficiently focused on the review question (perhaps they examine effectiveness in an unusual patient group; or only explore a limited set of outcomes). Such studies may sometimes be excluded. Alternatively, some studies might be rejected because they were not prospective randomised control designs. Others might be unacceptable because, even though they were randomised, the methodology was in some other way flawed. Checklists exist which allow the methodological quality of primary studies to be assessed (Guyatt *et al,* 1993; Crombie, 1996) and these are frequently used to make decisions to include or exclude specific studies.

In moving from a broad set of primary studies to a tightly defined collection which will form the basis of the review, good reviewers will ensure that they have explicit and objective criteria specified in advance to determine whether particular studies are to be included or not. In this way they try to minimise any bias which might occur from the selective inclusion of (for example) favourable studies. The impact of excluding studies of peripheral interest or methodologically dubious trials can and should be assessed in a sensitivity analysis (*p. 132*).

Flawed aggregation

Once the set of studies forming the basis of the review is fixed, the reviewer tries to aggregate the findings across the different studies. A simple tally of studies finding benefit against those not finding benefit is inappropriate as this would not take into account the different size of individual studies: other things being equal, more weight needs to be given to the larger studies. A statistical synthesis is conducted taking into account the number of patients included in each individual study. The result is a single summary measure of the size of any treatment effect (usually an odds ratio) (see *Chapter 5*; and Davies *et al*, 1998). This is 'meta-analysis' and it can be achieved in various ways (it may even involve the retrieval of individual patient data from the original trialists and a new full statistical analysis). The technical advantages and disadvantages of the various approaches sometimes employed in meta-analysis are complex and beyond the scope of this introductory chapter (Berlin *et al*, 1989). However, if the meta-analysis reveals only a small treatment benefit, there may be a need to examine more closely the reasonableness of the statistical techniques employed.

Heterogeneity

The original studies included in any review are always more or less a mixed bag: they will differ not only in the time and place of their execution, but also in the precise details of the patients included, the interventions received and the context of the delivery of patient care. The question is whether or not the extent of this diversity has material implications for the interpretation of the findings. This is largely a matter of judgement: although statistical tests to detect heterogeneity are frequently presented with meta-analyses, these are unable to detect anything except gross disparities between studies. Simple eye-balling of the individual study findings may be a more reliable guide to the presence of serious heterogeneity than an over-reliance on statistics.

If the studies included are considered too diverse, or the effect sizes described by individual studies appear widely heterogeneous, then there may be doubt over the wisdom of performing a formal meta-analysis in the first place. At the very least, any summary measure of benefit should be treated with caution.

Disguised fishing trips

Systematic reviews may cover many thousands of patients with diverse personal characteristics (demographic, clinical, social) seen in a variety of settings. When no overall effect can be demonstrated, reviewers can be tempted to go on a fishing expedition through various subgroups in search of individuals in whom the intervention is seen to work. Such findings, uncovered only in *post hoc* analyses, should be treated with caution bordering on downright suspicion:

> *If the fishing expedition catches a boot, the fisherman should throw it back, not pretend they were fishing for boots.*

> Mills, 1993

All subgroup analyses which were not clearly specified in advance (based on sound biological or clinical logic) should be seen at best as preliminary exploration requiring confirmation by future studies. Subsequent prospective studies may either provide such confirmation or demonstrate their deceptiveness.

Inadequate sensitivity analysis

Examining the data in different ways, especially the sensitivity of the findings to the decisions taken during preparation of the review, is an important step in establishing confidence in the results. For example, a sensitivity analysis might demonstrate that the findings are little changed whether primary studies of low methodological quality are included or not; or it might confirm that there is little difference in the results recorded in different health care settings (the United States *versus* Europe, for example). Sensitivity analysis can provide invaluable reassurance that the findings from systematic reviews and meta-analyses are robust. Such robustness refers to the stability of the findings even in the face of wide variations made in the review's underlying assumptions. Unfortunately, many reviews devote relatively little attention to this process, leaving the reader to wonder at the possible stability (and hence validity) of the findings.

Over-enthusiastic interpretation

It is in interpreting the numerical estimates of the effect size found in any meta-analysis that the most judgement is brought to play. Here the reviewers' natural inclination to have something to report may lead to an over-emphasis of supportive evidence and a comparative neglect of contrary data. In particular, we need to distinguish between statistical significance (relatively easily attained with the large numbers commonly seen in meta-analyses), and clinical significance (is the effect large enough to be worthwhile in clinical practice?). A further problem is that meta-analyses usually present their findings in relative (rather than absolute) terms, and this may influence judgements as to the importance of the effect (*Chapter 5*).

It is good discipline when reading a review to examine closely all claims made in the conclusions to identify the strength of evidence underlying them. In particular, unless the effects are large, or they are well supported by convincing and thorough sensitivity analyses, then some wariness in interpretation may be appropriate.

Generalisability and particularisation

Once assessed as robust, valid and sizeable, deciding whether or not the findings presented in a systematic review or meta-analysis can inform individual practice is, of course, a judgement for the individual physician. In making this decision the key questions to consider are:

- what patients were included in the review?
- in what settings were they treated?
- what was the precise nature of the intervention applied?

Only if the response to all of these is in agreement with local circumstances is adoption of the findings likely.

Conclusions

Systematic reviews are a major advance on the previous form of narrative reviews. Empirical work has shown that well-conducted systematic reviews with meta-analysis provide a reliable (but not infallible) guide to the effectiveness of health care interventions (Cappelleri *et al*, 1996; LeLorier *et al*, 1997; Crombie and McQuay, 1998). Discrepancies between meta-analyses and large randomised control trials have been seen (Villar *et al*, 1995; Cappelleri *et al*, 1996; LeLorier *et al*, 1997) and sometimes these have been serious (Egger and Davey-Smith, 1995). Nonetheless, 'clinically important disagreements without identifiable explanations are uncommon' (Cappelleri *et al*, 1996). Careful consideration of the basic principles on which unbiased review is founded, and the identification and assessment of any flaws therein, can protect health care decision-makers from having to take review findings on trust.

Further reading

A series of six articles in the *British Medical Journal* discussed the potential and pitfalls of systematic reviews and meta-analyses in considerable detail (Egger and Davey-Smith 1997; Egger *et al*, 1997; Egger *et al*, 1997; Egger *et al*, 1997; Egger and Davey-Smith, 1998; Egger *et al*, 1998). The interested reader will find both in these papers, and in a book by Chalmers and Altman (1995), much elaboration of the basic principles; they also provide a gateway to the burgeoning literature in this area. A number of published check-lists provide a convenient means of critically appraising systematic reviews and meta-analyses (Milne and Chambers, 1993; Oxman *et al*, 1994; Cook *et al*, 1995; Crombie, 1996).

Key points

* Systematic reviews with meta-analyses provide a good guide on clinical effectiveness but they are not infallible.

* Good systematic reviews include a complete set of all relevant and methodologically sound studies; the data from these studies are then combined in an unbiased and transparent manner.

* Problems may arise because: a) the review question is poorly conceived; b) the set of studies collected is incomplete or inappropriate; or c) the conclusions drawn are insufficiently warranted by the data presented.

* A detailed reading of any review can uncover flaws and allow assessment of the robustness of the main findings.

* Applicability of review findings remains a matter of clinical judgement not scientific exactitude.

References

Berlin JA, Laird NM, Sacks HS, Chalmers TC (1989) A comparison of statistical methods for combining event rates from clinical trials. *Stat Med* **8**: 141–51

Cappelleri JC, Ioannidis JPA, Schmid CH *et al* (1996) Large trials *vs* meta-analysis of smaller trials: how do their results compare? *JAMA* **276**: 1332–8

Chalmers I, Altman DG (eds) (1995) *Systematic Reviews*. BMJ Publishing Group, London

Cook DJ, Sackett DL, Spitzer WO (1995) Methodologic guidelines for systematic reviews of randomized control trials in health care from the Potsdam consultation on meta-analysis. *J Clin Epidemiol* **48**: 167–71

Crombie IK (1996) *The Pocket Guide to Critical Appraisal*. BMJ Publishing, London

Crombie IK, McQuay HJ (1998) The systematic review: a good guide rather than a guarantee. *Pain* **76**:1–2

Davies HTO, Crombie IK, Tavakoli M (1998) When can odds ratios mislead? *Br Med J* **316**: 989–91

Egger M, Davey-Smith G (1997) Meta-analysis: potentials and promise. *Br Med J* **315**: 1371–4

Egger M, Davey-Smith G (1998) Meta-analysis: bias in location and selection of studies. *Br Med J* **316**: 61–6

Egger M, Davey-Smith G, Phillips AN (1997) Meta-analysis: beyond the grand mean? *Br Med J* **315**: 1610–14

Egger M, Davey-Smith G, Phillips AN (1997) Meta-analysis: principles and procedures. *Br Med J* **315**: 1533–7

Egger M, Davey-Smith G, Schneider M, Minder C (1997) Bias in meta-analysis detected by a simple graphical test. *Br Med J* **315**: 629–34

Egger M, Davey-Smith G (1995) Misleading meta-analysis. Lessons from 'an effective, safe, simple' intervention that wasn't. *Br Med J* **310**: 752–4

Egger M, Schneider M, Davey-Smith G (1998) Spurious precision? Meta-analysis of observational studies. *Br Med J* **316**: 140–4

Guyatt GH, Sackett DL, Cook DJ (1993) Users' guides to the medical literature. II. How to use an article about therapy or prevention. A. Are the results of the study valid? *J Am Med Assoc* **270**: 2598–601

LeLorier J, Gregoire G, Benhaddad A, Lapierre J, Derderian F (1997) Discrepancies between meta-analyses and subsequent large randomized controlled trials. *N Engl J Med* **337**: 536–42

Mills JL (1993) Data torturing. *N Engl J Med* **329**: 1196–9

Milne R, Chambers L (1993) Assessing the scientific quality of review articles. *J Epidemiol Community Health* **47**: 169–70

Mulrow CD (1987) The medical review article: state of the science. *Ann Intern Med* **106**: 485–8

Oxman AD, Cook DC, Guyatt GH (1994) Users' guides to the medical literature: VI. How to use an overview. *J Am Med Assoc* **272**: 1367–71

Sackett DL, Haynes RB, Guyatt GH, Tugwell P (1991) *Clinical Epidemiology: a basic science for clinical medicine.* Little, Brown and Company, Boston: 380

Villar J, Carroli G, Belizan JM (1995) Predictive ability of meta-analyses of randomised controlled trials. *Lancet* **345**: 772–76

16

Reading and assessing qualitative research

Alison Powell, Huw Davies

What makes doctors burn out? What is it like to have epilepsy? Why don't smokers give up? Qualitative research makes it possible to look behind the statistics and to study health and health care from the inside: to find out what it is really like for the health professionals who provide the care and for the patients on the receiving end.

Many previous chapters have discussed why it is important for health care professionals and managers to be able to read and assess research reports critically, and have advised on how to carry out critical appraisal of quantitative research. This chapter looks at the role and benefits of qualitative research, and suggests how published reports might be assessed for their trustworthiness.

What is qualitative research?

Qualitative research aims to explore the meaning and not the frequency of social phenomena (Easterby-Smith *et al*, 1991). The assumption behind qualitative research is that the way individuals see and interpret the world, and in turn how they behave, is affected by their attitudes, beliefs and preferences. To understand human behaviour in a particular context, it is necessary to explore the individual's frame of reference and their definition of the situation. Qualitative research studies people 'in the field' (in their natural settings), and collects naturally occurring data (Bowling, 1997).

While quantitative research can tackle questions about the safety of a particular drug, or how often an event occurs in a given population, qualitative research can contribute to a richer understanding of health care by tackling the 'why' and 'how' questions. For example:

- why do so many student nurses leave training?
- why do some doctors oppose reductions in their working hours?
- how do the media affect public perceptions of the medical profession?

The distinctive methods of qualitative research make it particularly appropriate in certain research situations.

When is qualitative research used?

Qualitative research is useful when facing particular research challenges, for example, when the issue being studied is particularly sensitive or when little is known about it (*Box 16.1*). It can stand alone or can complement or supplement quantitative research. For example, it can be used as a preliminary step to explore what questions and choice of responses should be given to respondents in a questionnaire, or when constructing a scale to measure opinions. It can also be used to explore in more detail the issues raised by a survey already conducted (for example, why do 56% of respondents think that assisted conception should not be available on the NHS?). In tackling such issues, qualitative research uses a wide variety of data collection methods.

Box 16.1: What is qualitative research useful for?

Qualitative research can be used for:

❖ exploring new topics or areas about which little is known
❖ dealing with sensitive/complex issues
❖ generating hypotheses which can then be tested deductively
❖ describing in words rather than numbers the qualities of social phenomena, eg. caring for an elderly relative, unemployment, racial harassment
❖ uncovering the nature of an individual's experience of a phenomenon, eg. illness, bereavement, career transition.

     Derived from Strauss and Corbin, 1990; Bowling, 1997

Qualitative research entails:

... immersion in the everyday life of the setting chosen for study; values and seeks to discover participants' perspectives on their worlds; views inquiry as an interactive process between the researcher and the participants; is both descriptive and analytic; and relies on people's words and observable behaviour as the primary data.

     Marshall and Rossman, 1995: 4

Qualitative research methods

The specific data collection methods used in qualitative research will depend on the purpose of the research and on the type of question(s) being explored (*Box 16.2*). Of all these methods, the most commonly encountered are direct observation and interviews. There are several useful texts that describe these methods in more detail (Easterby-Smith *et al*, 1991; Marshall and Rossman, 1995; Bowling, 1997). Naturally there are specific pitfalls associated with each data collection strategy, but nonetheless it is possible to give general guidance to assist in the interpretation of qualitative studies.

Box 16.2: Methods of data collection in qualitative research

❖ Direct observation: participant observer or non-participant observer.

❖ Interviews: semi-structured or unstructured.

❖ Focus groups: loosely structured interviews with a small group and a facilitator.

❖ Repertory grid technique: constructing a mathematical representation of an individual's perceptions.

❖ Cognitive mapping: a variation of the repertory grid technique, used with groups.

❖ Projective techniques: exploratory techniques which use stimuli (eg. photos, drawings) to prompt individuals to 'project' their own meanings on to the stimuli and thus reveal aspects of their beliefs and feelings.

❖ Protocol analysis: seeking an individual's explanation of events shortly after an incident has occurred.

❖ Diary methods: structured or unstructured recording of events (eg. activities, symptoms) by individuals.

What to look for when reading and assessing qualitative research

One helpful way to determine the quality of a piece of research, and to assess whether its findings are worth further consideration, is to use a checklist to pose a variety of questions. As qualitative research is different in its nature and purpose from quantitative research, the kinds of checklists used to appraise quantitative research are unhelpful in assessing the quality of qualitative research. Because qualitative research has different aims and underlying assumptions, a different set of questions needs to be asked. For example, the common terms 'validity', 'reliability' and 'generalisability' mean different things when applied to quantitative and qualitative research and therefore the reader needs to ask different questions of each (*Table 16.1*).

Table 16.1: Questions of validity, reliability and generalisability		
	Quantitative research	**Qualitative research**
Validity	Does an instrument measure what it is supposed to measure?	Has the researcher gained full access to the knowledge and meanings of informants?
Reliability	Will the measure yield the same results on different occasions (assuming no real change in what is to be measured?)	Will similar observations be made by different researchers on different occasions?
Generalisability	What is the probability that patterns observed in a sample will also be present in the wider population from which the sample is drawn?	How likely is it that ideas and theories generated in one setting will also apply in other settings?

Adapted from Easterby-Smith *et al*, 1991

Set out below is a series of questions that could be used to assess the quality of a piece of qualitative research. The questions are given as a complete list in *Box 16.3*. The questions are derived from various sources including Bowling (1997), Gray (1997), Greenhalgh (1997), Mays and Pope (2000) and Silverman (2000).

1: Was the research question worth asking?

Research may be useful and relevant when it either adds to knowledge or reinforces what has already been learnt (Mays and Pope, 2000). It must also satisfy the 'so what?' test. The researcher needs to persuade the reader that the study, however small, was worth doing. It might, for example, look at a common and significant problem in clinical practice, or shed light on a new issue, or complement an existing piece of research.

The specific research question might not have been finalised at the start of the research: qualitative research can often be an inductive and iterative process (Greenhalgh, 1997) and the research question may be modified along the way as the data collected substantiates or disconfirms preliminary assumptions or hypotheses. However, in describing what they have done, the researchers should make clear their central research question(s), and the steps that led to this point.

2: Was the theoretical framework clear?

The report should make clear how the study fits in to an existing body of knowledge or theory. Did the study aim to test the findings of earlier researchers or apply theory in a new setting? For example, a case study of the introduction of new working practices for nurses in an outpatient clinic could be linked to theories about change management or build on theories about the operation of hierarchies in organisations.

3: Was a qualitative approach appropriate?

The nature of the research question determines whether naturalistic qualitative strategies were appropriate or whether quantitative methods should have been used instead. Testing the efficacy and safety of a new intervention would need quantitative methods while qualitative methods could be used to explore patients' attitudes towards the proposed new treatment. *Box 16.1* gives some indication of the areas of enquiry that are well-suited to a qualitative approach.

4: Did the methods used meet the needs of the research question?

The reader needs to have enough information to judge whether the specific data collection methods were a sensible and adequate way to address the research question (Greenhalgh, 1997). Good qualitative research is likely to use a variety of methods of data collection (and analysis). Triangulation compares the results of two or more methods of data collection (for example, interviews and observation) or from two or more data sources (for example, interviews with nurses from two different units), the aim being to make the data as comprehensive as possible (Mays and Pope, 2000).

5: Was the researcher's perspective clearly stated and taken into account?

The close involvement of the researcher can be one of the strengths of qualitative research as it makes it possible to gather a much more detailed and in-depth description of complex social experiences. For example, a skilled and sensitive interviewer can develop a good rapport with interviewees, which enables them to share information that would otherwise not be disclosed. The downside of this involvement is that there is a greater risk that observer bias will influence the results. This can work in both directions: the researcher may be predisposed to look for certain findings and the research subjects may themselves be influenced by the researcher's status (for example, if the researcher is one of the nurses caring for them). Good qualitative research builds-in strategies to balance bias in interpretation (Marshall and Rossman, 1995) and makes explicit the theoretical perspective and values of the researcher(s) so that the findings can be assessed accordingly.

6: Was the context of the research clearly described?

The researcher should provide information about the context in which the research took place: for example, the type and size of unit; how long the service had been running; any significant changes occurring at the time of the research (such as a merger of services or the development of a new programme). The timing of data gathering may also be relevant, for example, pre-discharge or post-discharge assessments from patients. This information is important so that the reader can both reflect on possible biases or confounding factors and relate the findings of the study to other settings. In qualitative research, generalisability is likely to be conceptual rather than numerical (Green and Britten, 1998), which means that the reader needs to be able to assess how far the findings and the theories developed (for example about patients' attitudes towards early discharge from hospital) could translate to their own specialty, type of unit or area of concern.

7: Was the sampling strategy clearly described and justified?

Good qualitative research often uses a diverse range of individuals and settings to increase both the validity of the account, (ie. its closeness to the truth; Greenhalgh, 1997) and the generalisability of the research (its value elsewhere). As such, qualitative research is not concerned with obtaining representative samples in the statistical sense: the objective is to look at why people behave as they do and not to estimate the proportion of individuals who hold a particular view (Crombie and Davies 1996; Marshall 1996). It is legitimate in qualitative research deliberately to seek out a group of individuals who fit the characteristics of the situation being researched (for example, health service managers who previously worked in private industry).

Three broad approaches to sampling have been identified: the convenience sample; the judgement/purposeful sample; and the theoretical sample (Marshall, 1996). The research question, and the type of data analysis envisaged, will determine the relative balances between these approaches — but convenience sampling alone (taking the first few individuals who happen to come along) is likely to lead to weaker accounts and limited generalisability. In all cases, the sampling strategies need to be made explicit so that the reader can judge their appropriateness.

8: Was the fieldwork clearly described in detail?

Data collection should be systematic and should be described in sufficient detail that it would be possible for another researcher to repeat each stage. Problems encountered during data collection (eg. refusals to participate leading to under-recruitment) which resulted in modifications to the original plan should be explained. Relevant documents (for example, a standard letter inviting patients to participate in the study) should either be included within the research report or be readily available.

9: Was the analysis convincing and replicable?

Methods of analysis of qualitative research are dealt with in detail in several texts (Strauss and Corbin, 1990; Marshall and Rossman, 1995; Pope *et al*, 2000; Silverman, 2000). The first key issue for the reader is: how systematic was the analysis? Was the coding of data carried out according to an explicit set of rules that clearly describe the categories used and the criteria for inclusion/exclusion? Is there sufficient evidence that the interpretation was based on the data and was not merely impressionistic or partial, with the investigator simply extracting and reporting on those data that supported their hypotheses (Bowling 1997)? Some authors suggest that the research report should contain enough of the raw data to help the reader to make this judgement (for example, Bowling, 1997) although, of course, this is difficult in short papers and it does not preclude selective inclusion.

The issue of whether or not more than one data collector and/or analyst should be used is debatable, and clearly has resource implications; however, multiple researchers may be helpful in situations where bias is particularly likely to be a problem (Pope *et al*, 2000).

10: How adequate was the discussion?

The discussion should set out clearly how the links were made between data, theories and conclusions. The reader needs to decide how well the analysis succeeded in incorporating the observations, for example, whether there was adequate discussion of the evidence for and against the researcher's arguments, and whether sufficient attention was given to the analysis of deviant cases (those that appear to contradict the emerging explanations; Mays and Pope, 2000). Finally, the discussion should acknowledge any limitations of the study.

Box 16.3: Checklist of issues to consider when reading qualitative research

1. Was the research question worth asking?

2. Was the theoretical framework clear?

3. Was a qualitative approach appropriate?

4. Did the methods used meet the needs of the research question?

5. Was the researcher's perspective clearly stated and taken into account?

6. Was the context of the research clearly described?

7. Was the sampling strategy clearly described and justified?

8. Was the fieldwork clearly described in detail?

9. Was the analysis convincing and replicable?

10. How adequate was the discussion?

Conclusions

Qualitative research can add much to a broad understanding of health care. It is different in both form and intent from quantitative research, and critically appraising it can be more difficult. Asking a series of key questions can help readers to assess the quality of a piece of qualitative research and whether or not to apply its findings in their own practice.

Key points

* Qualitative research, like any research, should be assessed for its trustworthiness (internal validity) and its generalisability (external validity).

* Qualitative research seeks to go beyond and behind surface descriptions of phenomena; to describe and explain phenomena from the participants' perspectives and from within naturalistic contexts.

* Qualitative methods are diverse, and each has particular strengths, areas of application and pitfalls.

* Because of the different intent and nature of qualitative research, different criteria for assessment should be applied than those usually used for quantitative methodologies.

* Engagement with ten questions (*Box 16.3*) can greatly assist a structured critical appraisal of published qualitative research.

References

Bowling A (1997) *Research Methods in Health: Investigating Health and Health Services*. Open University Press, Buckingham.

Crombie IK, Davies HTO (1996) *Research in Health Care: Design, Conduct and Interpretation of Health Services Research*. John Wiley, Chichester

Easterby-Smith M, Thorpe R, Lowe A (1991) *Management Research: An Introduction*. Sage Publications, London

Gray JAM (1997) *Evidence-based Healthcare: How to Make Health Policy and Management Decisions*. Churchill Livingstone, Edinburgh

Green J, Britten N (1998) Qualitative research and evidence-based medicine. *Br Med J* **316**: 1230–2

Greenhalgh T (1997) *How to Read a Paper: The basics of evidence-based medicine*. BMJ Publishing Group, London

Marshall C, Rossman G (1995) *Designing Qualitative Research*. Sage Publications, Thousand Oaks

Marshall MN (1996) Sampling for qualitative research. *Fam Pract* **13**: 522–5

Mays N, Pope C (2000) Assessing quality in qualitative research. *Br Med J* **320**: 50–2

Pope C, Ziebland S, Mays N (2000) Analysing qualitative data. *Br Med J*
320: 114–6
Silverman D (2000) *Doing Qualitative Research: A Practical Handbook.*
Sage Publications, London
Strauss A, Corbin, J (1990) *Basics of Qualitative Research: Grounded
Theory Procedures and Techniques.* Sage Publications, Newbury
Park

17

Aiding clinical decisions with decision analysis

Manouche Tavakoli, Huw Davies, Richard Thomson

As clinical decision-making gets ever more complex, new analytic approaches are being developed to assist. Decision-analytic models are used to structure complex decision problems in an uncertain environment by systematically linking decision choices with expected outcomes. Such models include the probabilities of outcomes and can also include patients' preferences, costs or both. These models can help to advise about therapeutic avenues. This chapter examines the nature of decision-analytic models, explains the reasons for their use, and explores the pitfalls in their interpretation.

Clinicians face many complex decisions in diagnosing and treating patients. Most diagnostic procedures provide not certainty but probabilistic information about the likelihood of disease. Treatments likewise may change the expected frequency of outcomes (desired or unwanted) but rarely offer guaranteed results. In addition, patients may have strong (but not always expressed) preferences regarding treatment strategies as well as their resultant outcomes. These preferences could and should be taken into account. It is under such manifold difficulties that doctors and their patients must make choices about diagnostic and treatment strategies.

Clinical research provides information that can feed into decisions about treatment strategies. Epidemiological follow-up studies can tell what happens to patients in the long term. Trial data can show the difference that interventions can make on a range of health outcomes. Patient preference studies can establish the utilities (values) that patients attach to certain health states. Combining and integrating information from all of these studies can help answer the question, 'which treatment strategy is most likely to bring the most benefit to the patient?' Often, integrating information from research studies into clinical decision-making is an informal process carried out by doctor and patient during the physician-patient encounter. Practitioners of evidence-based medicine may be more explicit in quantifying risks and benefits (Sackett *et al*, 1997) but this usually relates to clarifying the impact of a single intervention. However, for more complex decision problems, explicit analytic methods (called decision analyses) are available to assist. Decision analysis (DA) is an approach to structuring multi-layered problems and analysing the likely outcomes, benefits and costs from making certain decision choices. Investigations of clinical decisions using the techniques are beginning to appear in print, and such analyses can be used to underpin clinical guidelines.

This chapter explains the rationale for a decision-analytic approach and explores the main features of the technique. We highlight the advantages of the approach as well as expose some of the common pitfalls that may arise in using and interpreting the findings.

When is decision analysis appropriate?

Decision analysis may be appropriate when three factors come together: complexity, uncertainty and imperfect information. Each of these is explored below. Crucially, in many clinical decision problems it is the presence of all three of the factors which so clouds the decision choice.

Complexity

Technological and pharmacological advances in recent decades have presented clinicians with a far greater range of diagnostic and treatment options than hitherto. Clinical decisions may not be limited to a simple 'this or that' choice. They may be linked in chains where a decision at one point simply leads to another series of choices further down the line. For example, consider a patient with a hip prosthesis complaining of pain and with signs of infection. Should the patient be treated medically or surgically? If surgically, should the prosthetic replacement be done in a one-stage or a two-stage procedure? What use then of antibiotics? Which drug or combinations and by what route of administration? With this level of complexity, it may be difficult to assess the ideal course of action.

A second problem is the potential for trade-offs between different outcomes. Patients may have divergent preferences in how they trade-off gains in one outcome against losses in another. For example, the choice between radiotherapy and surgery for throat cancer may involve sacrificing life expectancy for increased quality of life. Making a decision requires striking a balance between various desirable outcomes and the unpleasantness associated with some treatments, with the knowledge that for some decisions there can be no going back (eg. in the case of surgery).

Uncertainty

In medicine the relationships between actions and outcomes are usually probabilistic rather than deterministic. There is always a chance that a good decision may turn into a poor outcome (or vice versa) even if the problem is well understood. Any analysis of a decision needs to manipulate probabilities rather than certainties. Such manipulations may be non-intuitive. Further, some individuals may be more 'risk averse' (disinclined to take chances) than others. The attitudes of the participants to risk have to be taken into account in order to arrive at an optimal decision.

Imperfect information

For all the burgeoning clinical research base, much remains unclear about the full implications of treatment decisions. The links between interventions and the complete range of outcomes may not have been established in all patient groups. In addition, the doctor may know little about patient preferences, either for outcomes (how do they value health improvements? how do they feel about side-effects?) or processes (how averse to surgery are they? do they value keeping their options open?). Decisions must be made with only an incomplete picture. Furthermore, even in the unusual situation where all the necessary information is available, there remains the problem that the human mind may not be able to integrate effectively such complex information.

The decision-analytic approach

Many clinical decisions are not supported by clear evidence such as a randomised control trial directly comparing the treatment options. Nonetheless, decisions still have to be made. Decision analysis is an attempt to assist in this process. It is an approach to structuring a decision problem so that decisions are related to outcomes in an explicit manner. It incorporates and helps identify sources of uncertainty, and presents this uncertainty in a quantitative way using probabilities. Once the problem is structured and tagged with data, it then becomes possible to analyse the expected outcomes (and, if necessary, costs also) for any given set of decision choices.

There are five basic steps to a decision analysis (Clemen, 1996; Drummond *et al*, 1994; Petitti, 1994):

1. *Identifying and bounding the problem.* This involves identifying the set of decisions under study, and listing the full range of possible outcomes. By carefully considering all aspects of the problem (including the aims and preferences of patients and health professionals) alternatives that were not so obvious at the outset (such as 'do nothing') might be uncovered and considered explicitly.

2. *Structuring the problem.* The aim is to simplify the problem by breaking it down into its component parts. The full range of outcomes which may flow from any decisions are identified, together with any further decisions which may then need to be taken. The aim is to develop a tree structure that flows from decisions (branch points) along various routes to different outcomes. The resulting structure provides clear linkages between decisions and outcomes. These are called decision trees, and an example is shown in *Figure 17.1*.

3. *Adding information.* A decision tree is a representation of the decision problem. However, before the tree can be analysed, it needs to be completed by adding in some quantitative information. These are the probabilities of the various outcomes at each stage of treatment, and the values that patients attach to these outcomes. Such information may come from a variety of sources, such as randomised control trials, observational studies, meta-analyses and reviews, new primary data collection and/or expert consensus.

4. *Analysis of expected benefits.* Analysis is done by a method of 'folding back and averaging'. That is, the 'expected value' of each decision choice is calculated from the probabilities assigned to the pathways and the utilities attached to the outcomes reached by those routes. This is done to determine the best strategy for the problem in hand, for example, to identify the route to the best likely outcome, or to the best cost-utility ratio depending on the stakeholders' objectives.

5. *Sensitivity analysis.* The complexity involved in decision trees may mean that small shifts in the individual probability estimates, or in the values (eg. utilities or costs) applied to outcomes, can lead to large changes in the likely optimal decision. Sensitivity analysis is the process of repeatedly analysing the tree using different values for probability and utility variables. The robustness of the conclusions from the model can then be assessed on the basis of variations in the expected values.

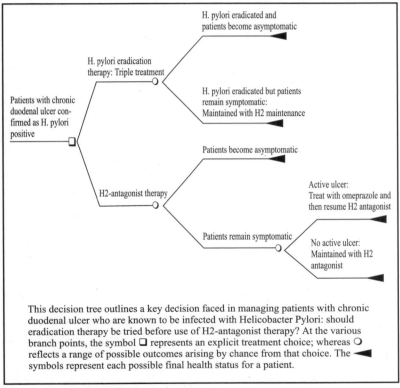

This decision tree outlines a key decision faced in managing patients with chronic duodenal ulcer who are known to be infected with Helicobacter Pylori: should eradication therapy be tried before use of H2-antagonist therapy? At the various branch points, the symbol ❑ represents an explicit treatment choice; whereas ❍ reflects a range of possible outcomes arising by chance from that choice. The ◀ symbols represent each possible final health status for a patient.

Figure 17.1: A decision tree

Decision analysis as an aid to decision-making

Clinicians cannot be expected to develop formal decision models when faced with making individual patient decisions. Yet decision-analytic models are appearing more frequently now in the literature and these can be used to inform day-to-day clinical practice. If this is so, then some grasp of the relative strengths and weaknesses of decision-analytic techniques is necessary so that clinicians can be discerning consumers of the information offered.

Decision-analytic techniques can be used to guide the management of individual patients or can be used to address policy questions about the use of treatments for groups of patients (Lilford *et al*, 1998). At present few models are available that can be customised to individual patient decisions (although the technology is available). More usually, DA models are used to clarify which treatment options are best on aggregate for patients with a given set of characteristics.

DA offers a number of advantages over more informal and intuitive attempts at synthesising a mass of complex data. Foremost among these are:

❖ *Clarity and quantification*. DA can clarify the extent of a decision problem through a thorough, logical and quantitative evaluation of alternative strategies. It makes the linkages between actions and outcomes (both good and bad) clear and explicit.

❖ *Consideration of preferences and costs*. Stakeholders' objectives and preferences can be modelled explicitly in DA models. Costs can also be included if desired.

❖ *Explicit trade-offs*. In some randomised trials the optimal decision remains uncertain because there may be several outcomes — and although the intervention may reduce the risk of one event it may increase the risk of others. DA can incorporate these trade-offs taking into account the patient characteristics which lead to different levels of risk (Naglie and Detsky, 1992; Lilford *et al*, 1998).

❖ *Exploration of options*. DA can facilitate exploration of a series of 'What if... ?' questions to allow a deeper understanding of the interconnectedness of decisions and outcomes.

❖ *Openness*. In DA, the problem is defined explicitly. This allows critics to identify parts of the model or underlying assumptions with which they disagree. This fosters clear communication and rational debate as to the model validity and, in turn, may bring about better conceptualisations and, ultimately, better decision-making.

Pitfalls in decision analysis

Like any research technique DA is not without its limitations. A good decision analysis may help inform clinical decisions but it cannot replace human input. In particular, any DA model is only as good as the data on which it is based. A number of potential pitfalls are described below together with suggestions for their avoidance.

❖ *The boundaries of the problem may miss important features.* One of the aims of DA is to focus the problem. Consequently the problem definition might omit important decision options (for example, 'watchful waiting') or may fail to consider all possible outcomes (for example, rare but disastrous side-effects). However, the explicit nature of decision analysis leaves such omissions open to scrutiny, and the question is not whether any particular DA is truly complete but whether its coverage makes it appropriate for the decision under examination.

❖ *Probabilities of different outcomes are only estimates.* These probabilities may be derived from either published literature or may simply be best guesses. As such, there may be considerable doubt as to the accuracy of these estimates. Good sensitivity analyses, which assess the robustness of the model conclusions to variations in these values, may help to reassure.

❖ *Expected benefits are benefits on average.* The purported benefits from any decision are expected benefits in the statistical sense only. That is, any individual patient may benefit completely or not at all. Expected benefits could be the result of a small gain for everyone or a mixture of large gains for some and losses for others. That is, aggregation inevitably averages out the experiences of both winners and losers, and DAs yield only this average value.

❖ *Patient preferences are usually in aggregate.* Although it would be possible to tailor a DA model to an individual using his/her own personal preferences, in practice this is problematic and rarely done. The patient preferences included are usually only incorporated in aggregate. Thus the recommendations from DA models may mislead if any individual patient has very different preferences from the group mean (for example, a very strong aversion to side-effects may override any expected benefits from therapy).

❖ *Estimating utilities for patient preferences is inexact and contentious.* Various methods are used to measure utility but none is fully established. The major problem is that different techniques can give diverse and at times conflicting results. Further, individual preferences may vary with time or experience, which may not be reflected in the analysis (Krahn *et al*, 1994). The most popular methods of measuring utility are standard gamble (SG) (Feeny and Torrance, 1989; Torrance ,1987), health utility index (HUI) (Boyle *et al*, 1995, Torrance *et al*, 1996), and time-trade-off (TTO) (Torrance *et al*, 1972; Torrance, 1987). This part of any DA model may need special examination and assessment. However, the standard gamble technique is generally considered to be the most reliable method of utility measurement (Feeny and Torrance, 1989; Torrance, 1987). It is based on expected utility theory, and it is the only method with an underlying theoretical base and so it could be argued that this should be the gold standard in the setting of DA.

❖ *DA models tend to focus on health outcomes and ignore process utilities.* Patients may gain benefits simply from having treatments even when no good outcomes accrue. For example, participants in assisted conception programmes may value the experience even if they do not conceive. Conversely, patients may fear and dislike surgery even when it produces good outcomes; and other treatment avenues may make considerable demands on patients in terms of clinic visits, monitoring etc. Patients may gain or lose utility from factors other than simply their health outcomes — and not all DA models take these factors into account. Finally, patients (and doctors) may value the ability to keep treatment strategies under review — whereas certain decisions preclude this possibility (a decision to proceed with surgery offers no possibilities of going back, while drug therapies may offer more flexibility). Because DA focuses on net expected values based on health states, it does not usually take into account the utility gained or lost in the processes of care.

❖ *Measurement of benefits and costs may contain hidden assumptions.* DA models which look at benefit/cost ratios may use differing assumptions in estimating either or both of these two quantities. Exploration of these assumptions is needed to reassure that they are reasonable. *Chapters 8* and *9* provide some advice on this.

Conclusions

Decision analysis (DA) offers a formal and structured approach to integrating large amounts of complex and probabilistic data. As such it can clarify decision problems, quantify (on aggregate) the benefits or otherwise of certain decisions, and incorporate both costs and patient preferences. Good DA models do this in an open and explicit way, using sensitivity analyses to explore the robustness of their recommendations. Nonetheless, DA models are complex to construct, contain many assumptions and make heavy demands on empirical data. Because of these limitations, DA models require careful appraisal and remain simply an aid to decision-making not a substitute for human judgement.

Key points

* Clinical decision-making is hampered by the complexity of the decision problems, the inherent uncertainty in the links between interventions and outcomes, and the incompleteness of the data available to inform choices.

* Decision-analytic models structure decision problems using decision trees and thus link choices to expected outcomes.

* Decision-analytic models offer advantages over informal assimilation of data in that they are open, explicit, structured, logical and quantitative.

* Decision-analytic models can be extended by including patient preferences (utilities) attached to potential health outcomes. They can also include costs.

* Decision-analytic models may still mislead if they are conceptually incomplete or are based on poor empirical data.

* Decision-analytic models provide recommendations based on the aggregation of expected costs and benefits, whereas actual clinical decisions are applied to individuals. Thus care is needed when particularising the findings from decision models to the care of individuals.

* Good sensitivity analyses can do much to bolster confidence in the robustness of the recommendations that emerge from decision-analytic models.

References

Boyle MH, Furlong W, Feeny D, Torrance GW, Hatcher J (1995)
Reliability of the Health Utilities Index—Mark III used in the 1991
cycle 6 Canadian General Social Survey Health Questionnaire. *Qual
Life Res* **4**: 249–57

Clemen RT (1996) *Making Hard Decisions: An Introduction to Decision
Analysis*. Duxbury Press, London

Drummond MF, Stoddart GL, Torrance GW (1994) *Methods for the
Economic Evaluation of Health Care Programmes*. Oxford
University Press, Oxford

Feeny DH, Torrance GW (1989) Incorporating utility-based
quality-of-life assessment measures in clinical trials. Two examples.
Med Care **27**: S190–204

Krahn MD, Mahoney JE, Eckman MH *et al* (1994) Screening for prostate
cancer: a decision-analytic view. *JAMA* **272**: 781–6

Lilford RJ, Pauker SG, Braunholtz DA, Chard J (1998) Getting research
findings into practice: Decision analysis and the implementation of
research findings. *Br Med J* **317**: 405–409

Naglie IG, Detsky AS (1992) Treatment of chronic non-valvular atrial
fibrillation in the elderly: a decision analysis. *Med Decis Making* **12**:
239–49

Petitti D (1994) *Meta-Analysis, Decision Analysis, and Cost-Effectiveness
Analysis: Methods for Quantitative Synthesis in Medicine*. Oxford
University Press, Oxford

Sackett DL, Richardson WS, Rosenberg W, Haynes RB (1997) *Evidence-
based Medicine: how to practice and teach EBM*. Churchill
Livingstone, London

Torrance GW (1987) Utility approach to measuring health-related quality
of life. *J Chronic Dis* **40**: 593–603

Torrance GW, Feeny DH, Furlong WJ, Barr RD, Zhang Y, Wang Q
(1996) Multi-attribute utility function for a comprehensive health
status classification system. Health Utilities Index Mark 2. *Med Care*
34: 702–22

Torrance GW, Thomas WH, Sackett DL (1972) A utility maximization
model for evaluation of health care programs. *Health Services Res* **7**:
118–133

18

Developing effective clinical audit

Huw Davies

Clinical audit received a mixed press when it was formalised as part of the health care reforms in the early 1990s — and has continued to mixed reviews ever since. Yet the latest governmental stipulations on clinical governance envisage a revitalised role for clinical audit. This chapter advises on avoiding some of the pitfalls that await the unwary in developing effective clinical audit projects.

Clinical audit has its roots in professional self-examination dating back to the early years of this century and beyond — even to the work of Florence Nightingale in the nineteenth century (Crombie *et al*, 1993).Yet it was not until the early 1990s that audit came of age, being included as a prominent part of the Thatcher-inspired health care reforms (Department of Health, 1989). The latest 1998 White Paper has reaffirmed the importance of effective clinical audit (Baker, 1998; Secretary of State for Health, 1998) and the demands of clinical governance should ensure renewed effort being devoted to the critical examination of the quality of local health care delivery.

Even from its inception clinical audit has had its critics (Maynard, 1991; Miles *et al*, 1996). More recent critiques have called for a refocusing of effort to ensure that audit delivers real quality improvements (Hopkins, 1996). This chapter addresses some of the key issues in the design and execution of audit studies, and advises on some of the steps to be taken to increase the likelihood of change flowing from audit projects.

Professional buy-in

Clinical audit often makes considerable demands on health care professionals over and above their clinical commitments. Any increase in workload needs to be accompanied by benefits perceived as commensurate. For health professionals, the benefits arising from audit are many and diverse (Robinson, 1996). Most obvious benefits include improvements in service delivery and insights into clinical practice, but also valued are enhanced professional standing, better communication with colleagues, improved knowledge and work satisfaction, publication opportunities or even promotion. Securing professional commitment to any audit project may be aided by paying attention to this broad range of professional pay-offs.

Of course, not all health care professionals are well disposed toward audit: many see it as boring, burdensome, time wasting and a distraction from patient care (Greenhalgh, 1992; Smith *et al*, 1992). Identifying and addressing such concerns is a crucial early task for those developing audit initiatives.

Although many individuals do carry out valuable audit projects, such single-handed projects can be unduly onerous and run the risk that a lack of multiple perspectives may lead to inadequate critical reflection. Developing projects in small groups has much to commend it, but brings in train the problems of increased complexity, co-ordination and (at times) problematic group dynamics. Multi-professional projects in particular are at risk of fragmentation and disintegration. The size and composition of audit project groups should, therefore, reflect the need for balance between including all the key players and maintaining the flexibility and dynamism seen in small groups. In particular, uni-professional projects, unfairly decried by some funders and commentators, may allow those with limited time and resources to side-step some of the difficulties experienced by multi-professional studies.

Clarity and focus

Many audit projects lack a clear purpose. Data on clinical practice are frequently interesting, and may be valued by clinical staff for a variety of reasons, but nonetheless can be ineffectual in securing change. It is the need to identify and implement changes in clinical practice which should lie at the heart of audit (Smith, 1990) — and other demands made of audit data should be subordinate to this overriding objective. Research shows that would-be auditors frequently struggle to 'close the loop' in the audit cycle (Mitchell and Fowkes, 1985; Mugford *et al*, 1991). A natural tendency is to think of data first and then speculate on how such data could be used (Crombie and Davies, 1991). A more disciplined approach begins with service change in mind and then examines the nature of the data needed to underpin such change.

Explicit standards

Defining explicit and objective standards has long been seen as a central part of audit (Fowkes, 1982). Yet many projects pay insufficient attention to this stage or even omit it altogether. This may be misplaced: clear thinking about the audit standards (with thorough references to established sources of evidence) may do much to focus audit activity and aim it squarely at practitioner behaviour change or service reorganisation.

Avedis Donabedian's classic categorisation of audit topics as 'structure' (the resources and facilities available for care), 'process' (the activities of care) and 'outcome' (the resultant effects on patients) still retains value in clarifying the nature of audit standards (Donabedian, 1968; Donabedian, 1988). Yet for all the recent emphasis on 'health outcomes', many local audit projects may be better served by focusing on the process dimension. Health outcomes by themselves can be difficult to collect and interpret (Davies and Crombie, 1997), and are insensitive to substandard practice (Mant and Hicks, 1995). Process measures in contrast are more readily collected, analysed and interpreted, and can direct attention at the core features of medical practice which need to be altered (Crombie and Davies, 1998). Crucially however, the advantages of process measures over outcomes are only seen when there is good research evidence to support the beneficial impact of those processes on important health status variables (Davies and Crombie, 1995).

Phased data collection

A second approach to focusing audit projects is to approach data collection in a phased manner and, initially at least, to pare back the amount of data collected to a bare minimum. In essence, audit seeks answers to a number of linked questions: is there a deficiency in current health care delivery? If so, why are things going wrong and what can be done to remedy matters? The data needed to answer these questions are as distinct as the questions themselves (Crombie and Davies, 1993). The first question lends itself to quantitative analysis of the patterns of care among substantial representative groups of patients (for example, analysis of the proportion of patients investigated and treated in a timely and appropriate manner). In contrast, the latter questions — answers to which are needed if effective change strategies are to be designed — may focus on in-depth qualitative analysis of a few cases to explore the underlying reasons for sub-standard care. Such an approach requires very different data collection strategies for the various stages of investigation. Yet too many audit projects conflate the two phases, collecting too much detailed clinical data from the outset, overloading projects so that they collapse under their own weight. Others neglect the latter phases altogether leading to poorly thought-out change strategies, ill-targeted at the underlying deficiencies (Johnston *et al*, 1999).

Problem-solving

That good audits are problem-solving in intent can be forgotten in the rush to collect interesting data. Yet audit data do not have to be watertight or generalisable to still prove useful. Audit is not research, which seeks to persuade others; audit is concerned with solving problems and bringing about local service change. As such, audit data need to be persuasive at a local level, clearly aimed at highlighting, unravelling and improving deficiencies in local service delivery. Imaginative audits may embrace mixed approaches on relatively small numbers of patients: quantitative analysis, qualitative study and even anecdote can all contribute to such problem-solving.

In order to achieve the primary goal of audit — effecting improvements in clinical practice — a key requirement is a clear understanding of the underlying problem (Crombie and Davies, 1993). Inadequate or incomplete understanding of this may lead to mis-targeted remedies. For example, many audit projects assume that clinical practice fails because of inadequate professional knowledge or ignorance of the failings. The solutions then sought usually embrace educational initiatives, guidelines and the feedback of comparative performance data. However, frequently the problems lie elsewhere: in lack of time, lack of resources, or patient pressure for example. In these cases, the feedback will be mis-directed and the impacts are likely to be few (Mugford *et al*, 1991; Bero *et al*, 1998).

Driving change

Accurate problem identification is only the start of developing effective change strategies (Johnston *et al*, 2000). Managing change is a complex and uncertain process, requiring attention to the many human factors that will either impede or facilitate change (Thornhill *et al*, 2000; Iles and Sutherland, 2001). First, changes need to be introduced with tact and sensitivity: audit can often imply a criticism of past practice that may be very threatening to established professionals. Second, there needs to be broad agreement within the clinical team about the need for change, the nature of that change, and the specific requirements that will bring such change about. Finally, some thought needs to be given to the potential resource implications and knock-on effects of change — otherwise losers in the system (or those who perceive themselves as such) may (consciously or otherwise) undermine the change strategy.

Technical support

Effective audits that tackle clinically worthwhile problems can pose significant difficulties during design, data collection and analysis. To experienced researchers, issues arising during data collection and analysis — such as questionnaire design, sample size and statistical inference — are familiar problems with well-recognised solutions. As the infrastructure supporting clinical audit and clinical effectiveness initiatives is strengthened, making use of this to ensure effective audits is only sensible. In particular, experienced audit facilitators may be able to offer much guidance and practical support.

Conclusions

For all the interest and money thrown at audit, results to date have been largely equivocal or even disappointing. Many projects have failed to deliver significant change to clinical practice — being long on ambition, short on resources and expertise, and diffuse in design. This does not mean that such projects are without value. Health care professionals report many and varied benefits from participation in audit projects even when no changes in clinical practice result (Robinson, 1996).

That audit has, to date, been limited in impact is perhaps unsurprising given the generally unstructured and *ad hoc* manner of its introduction. Wringing information from data is no simple matter, and changing health care delivery in the face of many forces of inertia is harder still. The experience of the 1990s has affirmed that such activities require skill and care, and frequently demand competencies from health care professionals that they lack. Experience from the United States shows a similar pattern of limited effectiveness from continuous quality improvement activities (Shortell *et al*, 1998).

Nonetheless, checklists and texts are available to support health care professionals as they develop audit projects (Bhopal and Thomson, 1991; Crombie and Davies, 1992). Thus, before the baby is dispatched with the bath water, properly resourced, well-focused and competent change projects built around the audit cycle should be given a chance to succeed. This will only happen when health care professionals develop the skills, and secure the support (financial, practical and attitudinal) needed for continuous service examination and change.

Key points

* Revitalised clinical audit will be an essential plank of clinical governance plans.

* Audits often fail because of insufficient attention to the underlying precepts.

* Effective audits are focused on delivering real service improvements.

* Explicit standards can help focus audit activity.

* Audit needs to move beyond describing potential clinical deficiencies and should emphasise identifying the reasons for these deficiencies and designing suitable remedies.

* Uncovering the underlying reasons for care failings may require imaginative and diverse data collection.

* Change strategies need to bring all the care team on board and should pay attention to the potential for change to be undermined.

References

Baker M (1998) *Making sense of the new NHS White Paper*. Radcliffe Medical Press, Abingdon

Bero LA, Grilli R *et al (1998)* Closing the gap between research and practice: an overview of systematic reviews of interventions to promote the implementation of research findings. *Br Med J* **317**: 465–8

Bhopal RS, Thomson R (1991) A form to help learn and teach about assessing medical audit papers. *Br Med J* **303**: 1520–2

Crombie IK, Davies HTO (1991) Computers in audit: servants or sirens? *Br Med J* **303**: 403–4

Crombie IK, Davies HTO (1992) Towards good audit. *Br J Hosp Med* **48**(3): 182–5

Crombie IK, Davies HTO (1993) Missing link in the audit cycle. *Qual Health Care* **2**: 47–8

Crombie IK, Davies HTO (1998) Beyond health outcomes: the advantages of measuring process. *J Evaluation Clin Pract* **4**: 31–8

Crombie IK, Davies HTO *et al* (1993) *The Audit Handbook: Improving Health Care through Clinical Audit*. John Wiley & Sons, Chichester

Davies HTO, Crombie IK (1995) Assessing the quality of care: measuring well supported processes may be more enlightening than monitoring outcomes. *Br Med J* **311**: 766

Davies HTO, Crombie IK (1997) Interpreting health outcomes. *J Evaluation Clin Pract* **3**(3): 187–200

Department of Health (1989) *Medical Audit: Working Paper 6*. HMSO, London

Donabedian A (1968) Promoting quality through evaluating the process of care. *Med Care* **6**: 181

Donabedian A (1988) The quality of care: how can it be assessed? *J Am Med Assoc* **260**(12): 1743–8

Fowkes FGR (1982) Medical audit cycle. *Med Educ* **16**: 228–38

Greenhalgh T (1992) Audit. *Br Med J* **305**: 961

Hopkins A (1996) Clinical audit: time for a reappraisal? *J R Coll Physicians Lond* **30**(5): 415–425

Iles V, Sutherland K (2001) *Organisational Change: A review for health care managers, professionals and researchers*. NCCSDO, London

Johnston G, Davies HTO *et al* (1999) Managing clinical audit: diagnosing the problems and designing solutions. In: Davies HTO, Tavakoli M, Malek M, Neilson AR (eds) *Managing quality: strategic issues in health care management*. Ashgate, Aldershot: 89–102

Johnston G, Crombie IK, Davies HTO *et al* (2000) Reviewing audit: barriers and facilitating factors for effective clinical audit. *Qual Health Care* **9**(1): 23–36

Mant J, Hicks N (1995) Detecting differences in quality of care: how sensitive are process and outcome measures in the treatment of acute myocardial infarction? *Br Med J* **311**: 793–6

Maynard A (1991) Case for auditing audit. *Health Serv J*, 18 July: 26

Miles A, Bentley P *et al* (1996) Clinical audit in the National Health Service: fact or fiction? *J Evaluation Clin Pract* **2**: 29–35

Mitchell MW, Fowkes FGR (1985) Audit reviewed: does feedback on performance change clinical behaviour? *J R Coll Physicians Lond* **19**: 251–4

Mugford M, Banfield P *et al* (1991) Effects of feedback of information on clinical practice: a review. *Br Med J* **303**: 398–402

Robinson S (1996) Evaluating the progress of clinical audit. *Int J Theory, Res Pract* **2**: 373–392

Secretary of State for Health (1998) *The New NHS — Modern, Dependable*. HMSO, London

Shortell SM, Bennett CL *et al* (1998) Assessing the impact of continuous quality improvement on clinical practice: what it will take to accelerate progress [see comments]. *Milbank Q* **76**(4): 593–624, 510

Smith HE, Russell GI *et al* (1992) Medical audit: the differing perspectives of managers and clinicians. *J Roy Coll Physicians Lond* **26**: 177–180

Smith T (1990) Medical audit: closing the feedback loop is vital. *Br Med J* **300**: 65

Thornhill A, Lewis P *et al* (2000) *Managing Change*. Financial Times, Prentice Hall, Harrow

Index